The
Mayo
Clinic
Diet

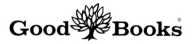

Intercourse, PA 17534 • 800-762-7171 • www.GoodBooks.com

Mayo Clinic

MEDICAL EDITOR-IN-CHIEF
Donald Hensrud, M.D.

ASSOCIATE MEDICAL EDITOR
Jennifer Nelson, R.D.

SENIOR DIRECTOR, CONSUMER PRODUCTS & SERVICES
Nicole Spelhaug

EDITOR-IN-CHIEF, BOOKS AND NEWSLETTERS
Christopher Frye

MANAGING EDITOR
Kevin Kaufman

CREATIVE DIRECTOR
Daniel Brevick

ART DIRECTORS
Stewart Koski, Paul Krause

ILLUSTRATOR
Kent McDaniel

PROOFREADERS
Miranda Attlesey, Donna Hanson

INDEXER
Steve Rath

ADMINISTRATIVE ASSISTANTS
Beverly Steele, Terri Zanto Strausbauch

Each of the habits in *Lose It!* has been the subject of scientific studies that support its role in weight management. In addition, Mayo Clinic conducted a two-week program to test the validity of this habit-based approach to quick weight loss. The 33 women who completed the program lost an average of 6.59 pounds, with individual results varying from 0.2 to 13.8 pounds lost. The 14 men who completed the program lost an average of 9.97 pounds, with individual results varying from 5.2 to 18.8 pounds lost. Individual results will vary. Consult your doctor before starting any diet program.

Good Books

PUBLISHER
Merle Good

EXECUTIVE EDITOR
Phyllis Pellman Good

ASSISTANT PUBLISHER
Kate Good

Published by Good Books

ISBN 978-1-56148-676-2

First Edition

If you would like more copies of this book, contact Good Books, Intercourse, PA 17534. 800-762-7171. *www.GoodBooks.com.*

For bulk sales to employers, member groups and health-related companies, contact Mayo Clinic Health Solutions, 200 First St. SW, Rochester, MN 55905, or send an email to *SpecialSalesMayoBooks@mayo.edu.*

The Mayo Clinic Diet is intended to supplement the advice of your personal physician, whom you should consult regarding individual medical conditions. MAYO, MAYO CLINIC and the Mayo triple-shield logo are marks of Mayo Foundation for Medical Education and Research.

Photo credits: Artville, BananaStock, Brand X Pictures, Daniel Brevick, Comstock, Corbis, DAJ/Getty Images, Digital Vision, Jordan Eady, EyeWire, Joe Kane, Rick Madsen, PhotoAlto, Photodisc and Stockbyte

Jacket design by Paul Krause

Printed in the USA

Table of contents

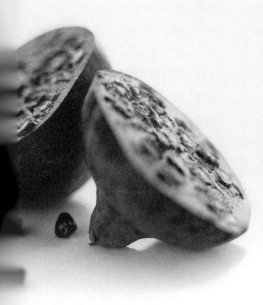

Table of contents (continued)

Introduction

If your experience is like that of many new patients I see, you've probably tried at least several diets in an attempt to lose weight, yet the weight keeps coming back. Welcome to *The Mayo Clinic Diet*, a program designed to be the last diet you'll need — or want.

This diet is not a fad. You've had enough of those and know the result. This is a program that helps you make simple, healthy, pleasurable changes that will result in a weight you can maintain for the rest of your life.

The Mayo Clinic Diet isn't a one-size-fits-all approach. Using clinically tested techniques, it puts you in charge of reshaping your lifestyle by adopting healthy new habits and breaking unhealthy old ones.

Why the emphasis on health? Well, Mayo Clinic is a medical institution, and good health is our goal. But aside from that, it turns out that a healthy lifestyle is also a great way to lose weight and keep it off. You get better health and better weight. Not a bad deal.

Perhaps best of all, this program is enjoyable. Eating is one of the great joys in life. What you eat on this diet has to taste good, or you won't do it. *The Mayo Clinic Diet* emphasizes foods that not only are healthy but taste great, which is why we can say, "Eat well. Enjoy life. Lose weight."

So dig in — turn the page and start today on a path to a healthier, happier life.

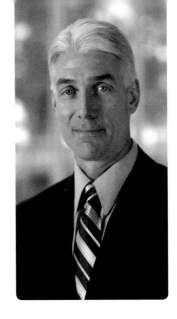

Donald Hensrud, M.D.
Medical Editor-in-Chief

P.S. Why did we write *The Mayo Clinic Diet*? Because you wanted it. Bogus Mayo Clinic diets — based on everything from cabbage soup to grapefruit to bacon — have been circulating for decades. These diets have no connection to Mayo Clinic, but their popularity told us that people are hungry for a diet based on Mayo's research and clinical experience. So, here it is — for real — *The Mayo Clinic Diet.*

How to use this book

This book is designed to help you start losing weight now.

Part 1, *Lose It!*

Jump-start your weight loss with a two-week quick start designed to help you lose 6 to 10 pounds in a safe and healthy way. Very little preparation — just read Chapter 1 and dive in. Part 1 is intentionally lean on background info because it's focused on *action*. Anytime you need more information, see Part 3 for additional help.

Part 2, *Live It!*

After *Lose It!*, transition into Part 2, *Live It!*, which is designed to help you continue to lose 1 to 2 pounds a week until you reach your goal weight — and then maintain that weight as you *Live It!* for the rest of your life. That's why there's no specific length for the *Live It!* phase of the diet — hopefully it will be a very long time!

Part 3, All the extra stuff

Part 3 of the book is all the additional information — meal planners, recipes, tips on overcoming challenges, and much more — that will help you understand the whys and hows of what you're doing in Parts 1 and 2, so that you can be successful in both *Lose It!* and *Live It!*

So, to use this book:

1. Jump-start your weight loss with Part 1, *Lose It!*

2. Continue losing weight and keep it off with Part 2, *Live It!*

3. Use the resources in Part 3 for help along the way and for more detail on the "why" and "how" of things, if you're interested.

4. While in *Lose It!*, look ahead to *Live It!* so that you know what's coming and can be ready.

5. While in *Live It!*, feel free at any time to repeat *Lose It!* if you want to boost your weight loss again.

Part 1 *Lose It!*

All you have to do to lose weight during this two-week period is:

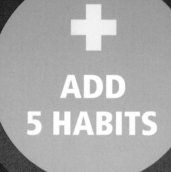

**ADD
5 HABITS**

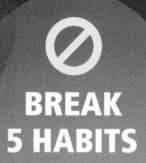

**BREAK
5 HABITS**

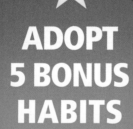

**ADOPT
5 BONUS
HABITS**

It's that simple. Get Started!

Chapter 1
Ready, set, go

You want to lose weight, so let's get going. *Lose It!* is designed to help you safely lose 6 to 10 pounds in two weeks and jump-start your weight loss. How much you lose is ultimately up to you — the more closely you follow *Lose It!*, the more you'll likely lose. This chapter provides some necessary preliminaries before you dive into losing weight in Chapter 2.

If you're overweight, you likely got there by having certain habits: Munching on chips while watching TV, ice cream before bed, maybe avoiding exercise. Often, people don't realize how much these behaviors, taken together, help pack on pounds. Habits — easy to get into, hard to break. *Lose It!* focuses on habits that affect weight loss.

All you have to do to lose weight during this two-week period is:

✛ Add 5 Habits
✛ Break 5 Habits
✛ Adopt 5 Bonus Habits

It's that simple.

To be honest, some of these habits may be challenging. No more TV time than time spent exercising? Eat breakfast — every day? You've got to be kidding. Actually, it's not as hard as it sounds — and best of all, it works (which you'll like). We'll provide tips and resources to help you succeed. And focus on this: By sticking to these changes *for only two weeks*, the pounds will come off, your health will improve, and you'll feel better.

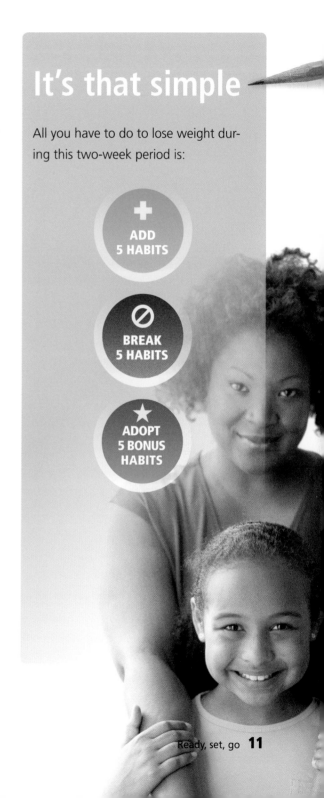

It's that simple

All you have to do to lose weight during this two-week period is:

+ ADD 5 HABITS

⊘ BREAK 5 HABITS

★ ADOPT 5 BONUS HABITS

Before you start

 Pick a start date. Before that date, familiarize yourself with the *Lose It!* habits and the tips on how to accomplish them. Make preparations. For example, one of the Add 5 Habits is to eat more vegetables and fruits. Good idea to have some on hand.

 On your start date, simply jump right in and begin following the Add 5 Habits, Break 5 Habits and Adopt 5 Bonus Habits. Page 19 directs you to helpful resources later in the book.

 Use *The Mayo Clinic Diet Journal* or a notebook to record your progress and track how well you follow the habits (see page 59 for an example).

 Use the Mayo Clinic Healthy Weight Pyramid on page 18 as a general guide to eating.

 Don't expect to be perfect (but try!). You'll likely have some slips, but the more closely you adhere to the habits, the better your results — and that's what you're after. When faced with a challenge, use the Action Guide to weight-loss barriers on pages 180-207 in Part 3.

 Pump yourself up for success. Use the motivational tips under *Yes, I Can!* on each page — or better yet, come up with your own motivators (see page 13).

Some of these habits may be big changes for you, but big changes bring big results. And remember, this phase of the diet is for only two weeks.

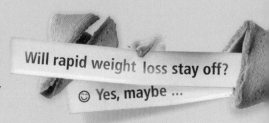

Will rapid weight loss stay off?

☺ Yes, maybe ...

Pounds lost through rapid weight-loss programs often come back — unless you make the necessary long-term lifestyle changes to keep them off. That's why there are two phases of *The Mayo Clinic Diet*.

Lose It! helps you see some quick results — a psychological boost — and sets the stage for *Live It!* It jump-starts those important lifelong habits that will help you keep pounds off and continue to your weight-loss goal.

The *Lose It!* habits are not intended to be followed as strictly in *Live It!* (although you can if you want to). The goal is to carry them over to *Live It!* in a general way, establishing a sustainably healthy lifestyle.

Finding your inner motivation

Odds are, you already have a pretty good idea of what you need to do to lose weight — eat less and move more. That's the basic calorie equation of weight gain or weight loss. But if you're reading this book, you probably haven't done it. Why?

Likely, you haven't found the necessary motivation.

Knowing the how-to, eat-this/don't-eat-that of weight loss is certainly important — and we'll help you with that. But the most critical element of weight loss is what *you* bring to the table — *your own personal drive to succeed.*

To be successful at losing weight, you need to figure out what will give you an *ongoing, burning desire* to succeed.

Throughout this book we'll sprinkle motivational tips and suggestions. They may help you think of things that you might not have thought of otherwise. Or they might serve as helpful tools when you're faced with challenges. But the best motivators come from within. How do you unlock your inner motivation?

Start by asking yourself this: "Why do I want to lose weight?" There may be several reasons. Improved health. More energy. Better beach bod. Whatever. Make a list of what's *important to you.* Then under each item write down specific reasons why it matters. **JOT IT** ▸

For example, let's say your top reason for losing weight is that you have a high school reunion coming up and you don't want to be embarrassed (OK, maybe that's not as important as improving your health, but let's run with it). Under that you write, "Show Bobby Jones (the boy who dumped you) what he missed," or "Not feel like a blimp on the dance floor." There are no wrong answers here — *it's what matters to you.*

Then find ways to keep those motivators in front of you — especially at moments of decision ("Do I eat that sweet roll or not?"). Maybe you use notes posted around your home and office, computer calendar reminders, or a photo of yourself as you want (or don't want) to look. Or write on the palm of your hand. Be creative. Just as you came up with your own motivators, use your own problem-solving skills to find ways to keep your motivation fresh and in front of you. The more the ideas come from you, the more successful you're likely to be.

It helps to be accountable

If you want to increase your odds of losing weight, get someone else involved. Involving others is a powerful motivator and can increase weight-loss success.

Enlist the help of a friend, co-worker or family member to be there for regular chats and support, maybe even a weigh-in. Or form a weight-loss group that gathers for a weekly weigh-in and meeting. Ask others to provide encouragement as well as accountability.

If you're unable to involve anyone else in your weight-loss efforts or you really prefer to do this alone, then at least be accountable to yourself — weigh in

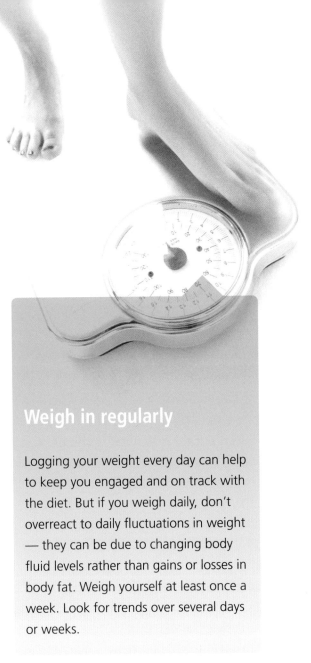

Weigh in regularly

Logging your weight every day can help to keep you engaged and on track with the diet. But if you weigh daily, don't overreact to daily fluctuations in weight — they can be due to changing body fluid levels rather than gains or losses in body fat. Weigh yourself at least once a week. Look for trends over several days or weeks.

regularly and record your weight in a journal. And regularly review your reasons for losing weight to help keep yourself on track. **JOT IT** ▶

Your starting point

Before you begin *The Mayo Clinic Diet*, determine your starting point: **JOT IT** ▸

+ **Record your initial weight.** Weigh yourself at a time and in a manner you'll be able to use consistently, such as right after getting up in the morning.

+ **Determine your body mass index.** BMI is a better indicator of body fat than is body weight. See the table on page 107 to determine your BMI. Write it down for future comparison.

+ **Measure your waist.** Use a flexible tape and measure around your body just above the highest points on your hipbones. Record your result.

You'll also want to:

+ **Consider your health.** If you have health issues, such as diabetes, heart disease, shortness of breath or joint disease, are pregnant, or have any questions about your health, see your doctor before beginning this or any weight management program.

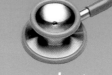

Talk to your doctor

Big changes in diet and exercise and rapid weight loss can sometimes lead to symptoms such as dizziness and fatigue or can necessitate changes in medications. If you experience these symptoms while on *The Mayo Clinic Diet* or are taking medications, talk to your doctor.

+ **Assess your readiness.** There's a good time to start losing weight, and there's a bad time. You don't want to put off your start date any longer than necessary, but you don't want to set yourself up for failure either by starting at a time when you're facing a lot of obstacles.

Answer the questions on the next two pages to determine if now is the best time to start a weight-loss program. If it's not, address those factors that are interfering with your plans to lose weight.

Once you've completed these steps, you're ready to roll. Review page 19 for helpful resources, and start following the habits in chapters 2 through 4.

Are you ready?

Circle one best answer for each question.

❶ How motivated are you to lose weight?

a. Highly motivated

b. Moderately motivated

c. Somewhat motivated

d. Slightly motivated or not at all

❷ Considering the amount of stress affecting your life right now, to what extent can you focus on weight loss and on making lifestyle changes?

a. Can focus easily

b. Can focus relatively well

c. Uncertain

d. Can focus somewhat or not at all

❸ Initially, people often lose weight quickly. But over the long run, it's best to lose weight at a rate of 1 to 2 pounds a week. How realistic are your expectations about how much weight you'd like to lose and how fast you want to lose it?

a. Very realistic

b. Moderately realistic

c. Somewhat realistic

d. Somewhat or very unrealistic

❹ Aside from special celebrations, do you ever eat a lot of food rapidly while feeling that your eating is out of control?

a. No

d. Yes

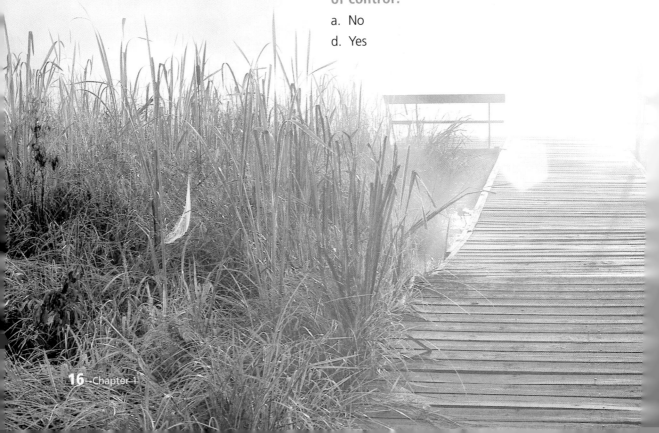

❺ If you answered yes to the previous question, how often have you eaten like this during the last year?

a. About once a month or less

b. A few times a month

c. About once a week

d. About three times a week or more

❻ Do you eat for emotional reasons, for example, when you feel anxious, depressed, angry or lonely?

a. Never or rarely

b. Occasionally

c. Frequently

d. Always

❼ How confident are you that you can make changes in your eating habits and maintain them?

a Completely confident

b. Moderately confident

c. Somewhat confident

d. Slightly or not at all confident

❽ How confident are you that you can exercise several times a week?

a. Completely confident

b. Moderately confident

c. Somewhat confident

d. Slightly or not at all confident

If most of your responses are:

+ **a and b,** then you're probably ready to start a weight-loss program.

+ **b and c,** consider if you're ready or if you should wait and take action to prepare yourself.

+ **d,** you may want to hold off on your start date and take steps to prepare yourself. Reassess your readiness again soon. You may want to talk to your doctor about what you can do to increase your readiness.

Note: If your answer to question 5 was b, c or d, discuss this with your doctor. If you have an eating disorder, it's crucial that you get appropriate treatment.

The Mayo Clinic Healthy Weight Pyramid

Throughout *The Mayo Clinic Diet*, use the
Mayo Clinic Healthy Weight Pyramid as
your guide to making smart eating choices.
There's detailed information on the pyramid
in Chapter 7 (pages 74-79) and Chapter 13
(pages 122-131), but the main message you
need now is to eat most of your food from
the food groups at the base of the pyramid
and less from the groups at the top, and
move more. Don't worry about being
too precise — just follow the general
pattern of the pyramid and you'll
be fine.

Sweets

Fats

Protein/Dairy

Carbohydrates

Fruits

Daily physical
activity

Vegetables

Quick reference guide to Lose It!

You can find answers to some of your most basic questions about *The Mayo Clinic Diet* on the pages listed here.

Basics

Healthy eating

Activity and exercise

Behaviors

Chapter 2
Add 5 Habits

The word *change* means many things:

→ To make different, amounting to loss of original identity (transform)

→ To make a difference that adapts to a new purpose (modify)

→ To break away from sameness (vary)

→ To make a difference without loss of identity (alter)

Add these 5 habits to your daily routine to make healthy changes.

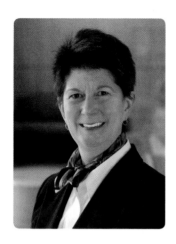

Jennifer Nelson, R.D.
Clinical Nutrition

When I talk with people about weight loss, it's important for us to explore what change means. Are you fearing the changes you think you need to make? Or, are you thinking that no matter what you do, it won't be enough to make a difference? I suspect that if you're reading this, you're somewhere in between. I want to reassure you that yes, you can change.

This is a fun chapter. Its focus is on adding good things to your routine. Yes, you'll begin each day by eating a healthy breakfast that will rev up your metabolism. Yes, you'll begin to eat more vegetables and fruit and switch to more whole grains — helping you feel full and giving your body nutrients it needs to rejuvenate itself. Yes, you'll find that healthy fat in small amounts keeps foods tasting great, while declogging arteries. Yes, you'll move more (and feel better).

Change doesn't need to be so drastic that you never try. We want you to meet change on your own terms:

+ Adopt a new purpose — you'll find that eating breakfast will set up your day for successful eating.
+ Break away from the same old thing — eating more vegetables, fruit and whole grains will fill you up, helping you stay away from calorie-laden foods.
+ Change your routine without losing who you are and what you like — become physically active doing what you enjoy.

No matter how big or small, these changes add up.

ADD 1

Eat a healthy breakfast

but not too much

What:

Have breakfast every morning. You don't need to eat a lot — just something to get you off to a good start.

Why:

Research suggests that people who eat breakfast manage their weight better than do people who don't eat breakfast. Breakfast is associated with improved performance at school and work, and it helps prevent you from becoming ravenous later in the day.

✚ Try whole grains, such as oatmeal, whole-grain cold cereal, whole-grain toast.

✚ Go for fresh or frozen unsweetened fruit.

✚ Low-fat milk and yogurt, an egg, nuts, seeds, and nut butters such as peanut butter can help you feel satisfied throughout the morning.

✚ If time is an issue, place a box of cereal, a bowl and a spoon on the table the evening before.

✚ Make a smoothie by taking fruit (bananas, pineapple, fresh or frozen berries), adding low-fat yogurt and blending to a smooth consistency.

✚ Hot or cold, choose your cereal by looking on the Nutrition Facts label for fiber (choose more) and sugar content (choose less). If you add milk or yogurt, choose reduced-fat or fat-free varieties. Top with sliced banana or berries.

✚ For French toast, dip whole-grain bread in a batter made of egg whites or an egg substitute, a pinch of cinnamon and a few drops of vanilla extract. Fry on a nonstick skillet or use a cooking spray. Top with thinly sliced apples, unsweetened applesauce, berries or sliced banana for sweetness.

+ Keep on hand food that you can grab and take with you to work. Convenient foods include apples, oranges, bananas, whole-grain bagels (mini-sized), pre-portioned cereals, low-fat yogurt in single-serving containers and low-fat cottage cheese in single-serving containers. Stir in berries or fruit to add fiber and sweetness.

+ Make a breakfast wrap with whole-wheat tortillas, roll in scrambled eggs with diced peppers and onions or peanut butter and bananas.

+ If you don't like traditional breakfast foods, look for something healthy that you do like. For example, fix yourself a sandwich made with lean meat, low-fat cheese, vegetables and whole-grain bread.

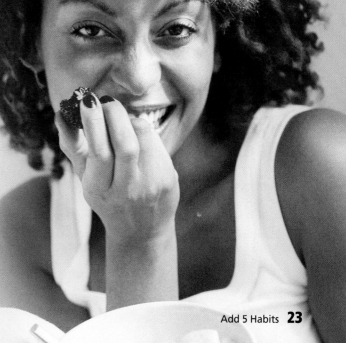

YES, I CAN!

If you're not in the habit of eating breakfast, start with just grabbing a piece of fruit as you walk out the door. Gradually include other food groups. Just like you got used to not eating breakfast, you can make eating breakfast an enjoyable and effective health habit.

If you don't eat breakfast, eventually your body says, "If you're not going to feed me, I won't be hungry," and you don't miss eating breakfast. But you'll overeat later in the day. Eating breakfast can help you lose weight and improve your health.

ADD 2

Eat vegetables and fruits

4 or more servings daily of vegetables and 3 or more of fruits

What:

Eat at least four servings of vegetables and three servings of fruits every day.

Why:

Fresh vegetables and fruits are the foundation of a healthy diet and successful weight loss. Most processed foods, regular sodas and sweets contain a lot of calories in just a small portion. Vegetables and fruits are the opposite — lots of bulk and few calories. You can eat generous portions while consuming fewer calories and feel full at the end of your meal.

HOW ↓

+ You don't need to like all vegetables and fruits — just some of them. Explore different types and varieties of vegetables and fruits for appealing tastes and textures.

+ Vary between raw and cooked vegetables. Lightly cook or steam them for softer texture. Sprinkle them with herbs for flavor.

+ Add a banana, strawberries or another favorite fruit to your cereal or yogurt.

+ When you're in a hurry, have ready-to-eat frozen vegetables handy as a quick addition to meals. Or use fresh vegetables and fruits that require little preparation, such as baby carrots, cherry tomatoes, cauliflower and grapes.

+ Vegetables, fruits and whole grains should take up the largest portion of your dinner plate. Eat these foods first, rather than reserving them for the end after you've finished other items.

+ When planning meals, think first of dishes that contain vegetables or fruits as the centerpiece and then build the rest of your meal around those.

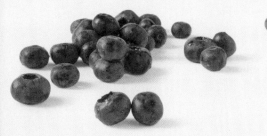

- Think fresh! Because dried fruit and fruit juice are higher in calories than fresh or unsweetened frozen fruit, the "unlimited servings" rule doesn't apply to them. Eating them could significantly increase your calorie intake.

- Snack on vegetables or fruits anytime.

- Look for ways to incorporate vegetables with other foods or into existing recipes. Add them to soups, casseroles and pizzas, and pile them onto sandwiches.

- Explore a local farmers market. The freshness and variety may encourage you to try new kinds of produce.

- When traveling, pack some ready-to-eat vegetables and fruits as quick snacks.

YES, I CAN!

On this program you have the green light to eat veggies and fruit whenever you want and as much as you want. Take advantage of it! Eat them first during a meal to make sure you get them in. Reach for them as snacks. If you're hungry — eat!

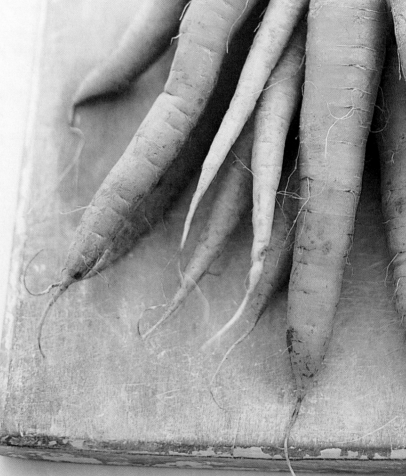

ADD 3

Eat whole grains

whole-grain bread, brown rice, oatmeal and others

What:

Focus on whole-grain breads, pastas, brown rice, oatmeal and other whole-grain products, instead of white, refined and highly processed products.

Why:

Whole grains include the entire grain kernel, which is packed with essential vitamins, minerals and fiber that are part of a healthy diet. Whole grains also fill you up by adding bulk, and they reduce your risk of being overweight.

HOW
↓

+ Eat whole-grain cereal, such as oatmeal or a bran cereal, at breakfast, or try whole-grain toast instead of white.

+ For ready use, stock your pantry with whole-grain breads (for variety, don't forget bagels and pita bread), crackers, and pastas, oatmeal, whole-grain brown and wild rice, and whole-grain cereals that aren't sweetened (if you want added sweetness, pile on fruit).

+ Prepare a meatless main dish such as whole-wheat spinach lasagna, red beans over brown rice, whole-wheat spaghetti with marinara sauce (see page 241), or vegetable stir-fry over brown rice.

+ Include a side dish using bulgur (see page 240), kasha, brown rice (see page 242) or whole-grain barley.

+ Try adding wild rice or whole-grain barley to soups, stews and casseroles.

+ Substitute half whole-grain flour for the white flour in pancake, waffle, muffin and bread recipes.

- When shopping for whole-grain products, look at the food label for specific ingredients such as whole wheat, whole oats or brown rice. Terms such as *100% wheat, multi-grain and stone-ground* do not mean the product contains whole grains.

- Use instant brown rice as a quick and healthy alternative to white rice.

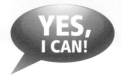

YES, I CAN!

Whole-grain products may taste different at first if you're not used to them. But if you give them a try, you'll probably learn to like them. Think about foods you didn't like when you were younger but that you like now.

Many people find that when they get used to the full flavor and texture of whole grains, it's hard to go back to their refined counterparts.

Go for the fiber

Grains (and fruits and vegetables) contain a kind of carbohydrate, called fiber, that resists digestive enzymes and can't be absorbed by your body. There are two main types — insoluble and soluble. Insoluble fiber — called roughage — is coarse, indigestible plant material best known for promoting healthy digestion. Many common vegetables and whole grains contain significant amounts. Soluble fiber — vegetable, fruit and grain matter that absorbs water — helps lower blood cholesterol levels. Barley, oats and beans contain notable amounts. Fiber-rich foods also slow the uptake of glucose, helping to keep blood sugar steady. Experts recommend consuming 20 to 35 grams of fiber a day.

ADD 4

Eat healthy fats

olive oil and vegetable oils, nuts

What:

When consuming fat, make healthy choices —
olive oil, vegetable oils, avocado, nuts and nut
butters, and the oils that come from nuts.

Why:

These fats are the most heart healthy. But
all fats contain about the same number of
calories, so even the healthier kinds should be
consumed sparingly to better manage weight.

HOW
↓

+ Check food labels. Compare similar
  foods and choose the one that's lower
  in fat (but make sure that it's also lower
  in calories — some low-fat and fat-free
  foods may be higher in sugar and not
  much lower in calories).

+ The types of fat in commercially made
  products are listed on Nutrition Facts
  labels. Reduce foods high in saturated
  fat and trans fat, and select more foods
  made with unsaturated fats (polyunsaturated and monounsaturated).

+ To reduce saturated fat intake, choose
  reduced-fat or fat-free milk, yogurt, sour
  cream, cheese and other dairy products.

+ Select reduced-calorie or fat-free dressings, flavored vinegars or oil-vinegar
  dressings for your salads. If you don't
  use reduced-calorie dressings, use a
  small amount of extra-virgin olive oil and
  vinegar (try balsamic, red wine and others). Sprinkle salads with a spoonful of
  slivered nuts or sunflower seeds.

+ Low-fat cooking techniques save unwanted calories. Try grilling, broiling,
  baking, roasting or steaming. A good-
  quality nonstick pan may allow you to

cook food without using oil or butter. You can also try cooking spray, low-sodium broth or water instead of using cooking oil.

+ Choose meat with the least amount of visible fat. Trim most of the fat from the edges of the meat. Remove all skin from poultry before cooking. Eat smaller amounts of meat (about the size of a deck of cards). Even small amounts of lean meat and poultry have fat.

Fats: The good and the bad

Monounsaturated and polyunsaturated fats are the best choices. Look for products with little or no saturated fats, and avoid trans fats — both increase blood cholesterol levels. Remember that all fats are high in calories.

+ Monounsaturated fats are found in olive, canola and peanut oils, as well as most nuts and avocados.
+ Polyunsaturated fats are found in other plant-based oils, such as safflower, corn, sunflower, soybean, sesame and cottonseed oils.
+ Saturated fats are found in animal-based foods, such as meats, poultry, lard, egg yolks and whole-fat dairy products (including butter and cheese). They're also in cocoa butter and coconut, palm and other tropical oils, which are used in many coffee lighteners, snack crackers, baked goods and other processed foods.
+ Trans fats — also called hydrogenated vegetable oil — are found in hardened vegetable fats, such as stick margarine and vegetable shortening, and in foods made with them (including many crackers, cookies, cakes, pies and other baked goods, as well as many candies, snack foods and french fries).

ADD 5

Move!

walk or exercise for 30 minutes or more every day

What:

Every day, include at least 30 minutes of exercise or walking in your schedule.

Why:

Eating provides calories. Physical activity burns calories. The more physically active you are, the more calories you burn. In addition, physical activity, including exercise, has many health benefits.

HOW
↓

+ The best exercise is the one you'll do, and the best time to exercise is whenever you can.

+ Any activity is good activity. Walking to the store, weeding the garden and cleaning the house all count.

+ Three 10-minute sessions of brisk walking can provide almost the same benefits that one 30-minute session does.

+ Make "excuses" to become more physically active. Include regular activity breaks in your day to stretch and walk around. Take the stairs instead of the elevator, at least for a few floors. Walk a few extra blocks from where you parked your car. It all adds up.

Instead of sitting down to watch television or check your email when you get home, put on your walking shoes and go for a walk. Watch your favorite program or read while you walk on a treadmill or pedal a stationary bike.

Make exercise enjoyable. Schedule time for exercise with a friend. Listen to music. Mix things up — don't feel tied to one activity.

If you haven't been physically active, start slowly and give your body a chance to get used to increased activity. A common mistake is starting an activity program at too high an intensity.

If you have trouble getting started, tell yourself that you'll exercise for only five minutes, then reassess. Chances are you'll keep going — and feel better.

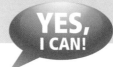

The hardest part about physical activity is not the doing but the getting started — putting on your shoes and getting out the door to walk or run. Psych yourself up with positive self-talk to overcome any hesitation when you're deciding whether or not to exercise.

Positive self-talk tips

+ Instead of, "I'm so tired," tell yourself, "I'll feel so energized when I'm done."
+ Instead of, "I should be better at this by now," tell yourself, "I've made real progress."
+ Instead of, "Skipping this one won't matter," tell yourself, "Every little bit makes a difference."
+ Instead of, "I'll never stick with this exercise program," tell yourself, "Take one day at a time."

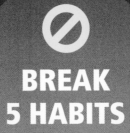

**BREAK
5 HABITS**

Chapter 3
Break 5 Habits

Changing any habit can be challenging. Changing a habit
that has been going on for many years, that involves our
emotional, social and psychological lives, is difficult. But
change is possible. Here are 5 habits to break that can make
a difference in your weight.

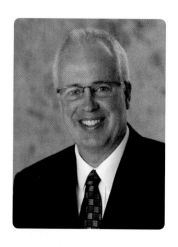

Matthew Clark, Ph.D.
Psychology

By using the right strategies for *you,* you can succeed in breaking the five unhealthy habits detailed in this chapter. Try these ideas:

+ Have confidence in yourself. If we believe in ourselves, we can succeed.
+ Anticipate urges and plan strategies for managing urges. If every day at work, for the past 10 years, when I'm under stress I've walked to the break room and had a candy bar, I shouldn't expect my desire for candy bars to just disappear. Having an urge is OK. Giving in to the urge is the problem.
+ When you get an urge:
  1. Tell yourself the urge will last for at most 20 minutes — just manage the next few minutes.
  2. Do something. Mentally distract yourself (call a friend, read a book), use positive self-talk (remind yourself of your goals), or physically do something (clean your house, take a walk).
+ Focus on what you're adding to your life. Many people losing weight have told me it often seems that they're avoiding doing things, like not eating ice cream. Sometimes, it can be more successful to focus on what I need to do, rather than what I'm trying not to do.
+ Use social support. Being around positive people that we care about can help us make changes.

Changing habits is challenging, but with confidence and the right strategies, you can succeed.

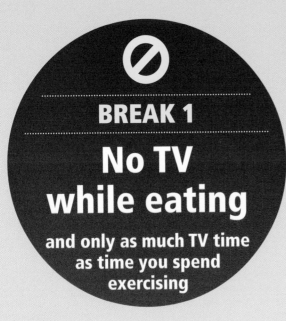

BREAK 1

No TV while eating

and only as much TV time as time you spend exercising

What:

Don't watch TV while eating (or, flipping it around, no eating while watching TV). Same applies for any "screen time," such as computer use. And, spend only as much time watching TV as you do exercising.

Why:

Studies show that watching TV contributes to increased weight — you aren't moving, and there's also a good chance that you're sipping or nibbling on something. If you establish the rule of no TV or "screen time" while eating, and only as much time watching TV as time you spend exercising, you're breaking one bad habit (mindless nibbling) while developing a good one (being more active).

+ Put a sticky note on the TV and the remote control to remind yourself that you need to exercise before watching TV or while watching TV.

+ Put a sticky note on your computer to remind yourself not to eat while using the computer.

+ Build up TV time by exercising before you turn on the set. Don't use TV minutes before you've earned them.

+ Turn the TV off while eating — you may be more likely to overeat if you get lost in a TV show and don't pay attention to how much you're eating.

+ Exercise while watching TV. The possibilities are limited only by your imagination.

Some ideas include:
→ Walking "laps" around the living room
→ Walking on a treadmill
→ Using a stationary bike
→ Marching in place
→ Doing calisthenics
→ Lifting weights
→ Using exercise bands

- If you're watching a longer program, exercise during the program and take recovery breaks during the ads, or vice versa if you're very new to exercise.

- If you're pinched for time, record programs and skip through the commercials when you watch later on. This can reduce watching time by about one-third.

- Record your TV time as you do exercise time, using *The Mayo Clinic Diet Journal*. The two times should match. **JOT IT** ▶

- Use a weekly TV programming guide to schedule exercise at the times when your favorite shows are on. There's no reason to exclude enjoyment while you control the amount of time you watch. Stick to your schedule once it's set.

- Skip the TV altogether and go outside for a walk, bike ride or run, or to do vigorous yardwork.

- Look for alternatives that help you break the habit of watching TV as you do other things. You're more likely to move more if you listen to the radio or to books on tape. Put on some music and move!

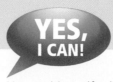

YES, I CAN!

Use positive self-talk — "I can do this!" instead of "I can't do this." Talk yourself up, not down. Focus on positives, not negatives.

- "Out of sight, out of mind," may be the best way to reduce the temptation of turning on the TV. Move your set so that it's not a focal point of the room.

- Watch TV at only one place in the house. Disconnect or remove all other TVs. In particular, TV sets located in bedrooms and kitchens can lure you into motionless watching.

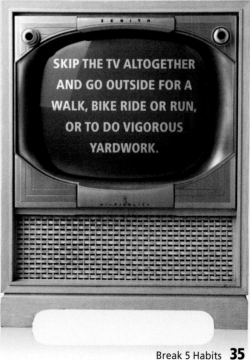

SKIP THE TV ALTOGETHER AND GO OUTSIDE FOR A WALK, BIKE RIDE OR RUN, OR TO DO VIGOROUS YARDWORK.

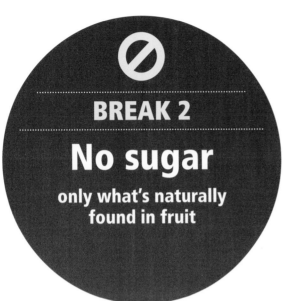

BREAK 2

No sugar

only what's naturally found in fruit

What:

If you want something sweet, eat fresh fruit. Otherwise, no sugar from common sources — candy, table sugar, brown sugar, honey, jam, jelly, desserts, sweets, and foods that contain more than a tiny amount of sugar or high-fructose corn syrup (such as soda and some coffee drinks).

Why:

Sugar has calories but no nutritional value. Sugar intake has increased tremendously in the United States over the past few decades and has contributed to the increase in obesity.

HOW
↓

+ Before you start the program, rid your home of sweets and sodas, stock up on fresh fruit, and replenish it regularly.

+ Keep fresh or unsweetened frozen or canned fruit available at home and at the office so that you've got healthy snacks available.

+ Instead of sugar, put fresh fruit on your morning cereal, toast, pancakes or plain yogurt.

+ Avoid cereals that contain sugar. Instead, try whole-grain cereals such as oatmeal, and use fruit and spices to enhance flavor.

+ Experiment with spices — try cinnamon in unsweetened applesauce as a spread on pancakes or toast. Other spices that may add sweetness include allspice, cardamom, cloves, ginger and nutmeg.

+ Read labels to look for sugar in products. If corn syrup, dextrose, sucrose, glucose, fructose, maltose, turbinado sugar, molasses or high-fructose corn syrup is listed among the first few ingredients on a label, the product likely has a high sugar content and should be avoided.

- Make your own fruit popsicles by blending one or more fruits with a little juice and freezing the mixture.

- Alcohol is counted as a sugar, and no alcohol is allowed in *Lose It!*

- Substitute fruit juice mixed with sparkling water for soda. Or make a fruit smoothie in the blender, mixing fat-free vanilla frozen yogurt and fat-free milk with fruit or frozen juice concentrate.

- Be creative and test your culinary skills. For dessert, prepare baked apples or grilled pineapple.

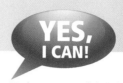

YES, I CAN!

To be successful, it helps to believe that you can lose weight and to visualize yourself accomplishing your goal. Believe it, see it, do it!

- Try new tastes that challenge and motivate you — and help divert your attention from more familiar, sugar-laden food. Serve fruits such as kumquat, lychee, mango, papaya, pomegranate, star fruit or Ugli fruit, which can be obtained at many grocery stores or specialty food stores.

Need to soothe your sweet tooth?

Why not just stock up on foods containing low-calorie artificial sweeteners? Sounds like a perfect solution, adding the sweetness of sugar without all the calories or carbohydrates. Not so fast! Many ready-to-eat foods using low-calorie sweeteners — such as diet sodas, candies and cookies — have little nutritional value and should be avoided. In addition, new studies have raised concerns that consuming foods containing low-calorie sweeteners may actually lead to increased calorie intake and weight gain (if you don't feel inhibited by the sugar, you may eat more than you would otherwise). Low-calorie sweeteners can be part of a healthy-eating plan — if they're used with care and in moderation. But in the two-week *Lose It!* phase, avoid sugar substitutes.

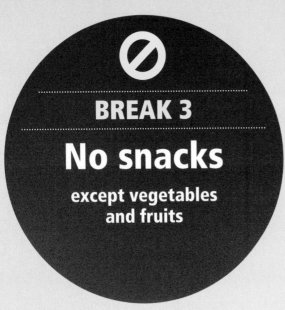

BREAK 3

No snacks

except vegetables and fruits

HOW ↓

What:

If you want to snack between meals, make it only vegetables or fruits and nothing else.

Why:

Common snacks typically have a lot of calories and little nutritional value for their volume. Vegetables and fruits are just the opposite — they can fill you up without contributing many calories to your daily total, and they're packed with healthy nutrients. Snacking can be a double-edged sword — snacking on vegetables and fruits a couple of times a day can actually help you manage your weight, while snacking on some conventional commercial snacks can pack on pounds.

+ Before you start the program, remove from your home all conventional snacks, including cookies, chips, candy and ice cream. Don't tuck them away in the back of a cupboard or freezer. Don't think you can resist the temptation of opening the package. Get rid of them! If it's in your house, it's in your mouth.

+ Stock your home with plenty of ready-to-eat vegetables and fruits. Don't expect to get by just on baby carrots — they should be one of many different options you can choose from.

+ Keep vegetables and fruits available at the office so they're handy for snacks.

+ Try a variety of vegetables and fruits so you don't get bored with one kind. For example, for fruit, instead of the familiar apples and oranges, try kiwi, mango, Bing cherries and apricots.

+ Experiment with sprinkling different spices and herbs on vegetables and fruits to create new flavors.

+ Establish a pattern of healthy eating every day. Space meals at intervals that are not too long. Allowing too much time to pass between meals can create a raven-ous hunger that drives you to mindless snacking.

+ Have some shelf-stable fruits and vegeta-bles at home, for example, unsweetened canned or frozen fruit, frozen vegetables or low-sodium vegetable juice.

+ If you're not in the habit of reaching for vegetables and fruits first, make an ef-fort to choose them anytime during the day, both as a snack and at the begin-ning of meals.

+ Identify situations that lead you to snacking, and then try to avoid them or find alternate activities. If you habitu-ally snack during work breaks, try going for a walk instead. If you can't resist a candy bar whenever you walk past the drugstore, find a different route. If emo-tions such as anger or sadness give you ice-cream cravings, call or talk to a friend who can listen and help relieve your urge to snack.

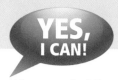

YES, I CAN!

When you feel like a snack, distract yourself. Grab a piece of fruit or some vegetables and go for a short walk.

+ Distraction is one of the best ways to get you past a snack craving. Prepare a list of enjoyable activities that you have at the ready for when a craving starts. Some form of exercise is an easy method of diverting your attention, but you can also pursue a hobby or enlist a family member or friend to contact for support.

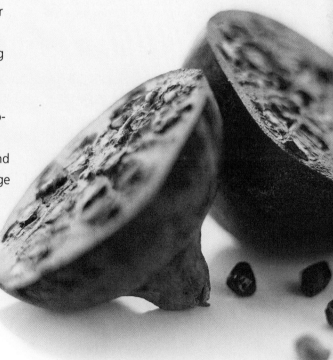

BREAK 4

Moderate meat & low-fat dairy

the size of a deck of cards and low-fat dairy

What:

Picture the size of a deck of cards (about 3 ounces of meat). Limit total daily consumption of meat, poultry and fish to that. In addition, if you consume dairy products, use only skim milk and low-fat products, and consume them in moderation.

Why:

Even lean cuts of meat and skinless poultry have some saturated fat and cholesterol and can be high in calories. And full-fat dairy products contain saturated fat that raises cholesterol.

Alternatives that are lower in fat and calories are available for both meat and full-fat dairy products. If you eat a variety of foods and get enough calories, you can get enough protein even on a vegetarian diet.

HOW
↓

+ Legumes and soy products such as tofu are excellent alternatives to animal sources of protein. A ½-cup serving of cooked beans, peas, lentils or tofu is about the same as a 2-ounce serving of meat, poultry or fish.

+ Use skim milk or low-fat yogurt and cheese instead of full-fat dairy products.

+ Don't make meat the focus of your meals. Instead, build the main part of your meal around vegetables, fruits and whole-grain rice and pasta.

+ Go for quality instead of quantity. Instead of a large piece of medium-quality meat, have a small piece of a good-quality cut.

+ Trim all visible fat from meat sources and remove the skin from poultry before eating.

+ Choose meat, poultry or fish that's roasted, broiled, baked or grilled rather than fried — and avoid any entrée that's breaded. The manner in which food is prepared greatly affects how much fat and calories you consume.

+ If buying ground turkey, buy packages marked "ground turkey breast" versus "ground turkey," which may have the skin added.

+ Include more meatless meals in your diet, including stir-fry dishes, casseroles, salads, and even sandwiches (generously stuffed with veggies).

+ Try whole-wheat pasta with tomato sauce and lots of cut-up broccoli, zucchini and bell peppers. Enjoy pizza with onions, peppers, mushrooms, tomato slices and artichokes. Or make a meal of red beans and rice, split pea or lentil soups, or meatless three-bean chili (with kidney, black and garbanzo beans).

+ Substitute baked or grilled fish for red meat — at least two servings of fish are recommended each week. Along with being lower in saturated fat than is meat, fish such as albacore tuna, salmon, mackerel, herring and sardines are high in omega-3 fatty acids that reduce your risk of cardiovascular disease.

+ Try veggie burgers or veggie hot dogs, which are often made with tofu, grains or vegetables.

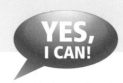

YES, I CAN!

Throughout the day you'll make decisions that affect how well you follow this program. "Do I eat a hamburger and fries or a salad?" "Do I go for a walk or not?" Be prepared for those moments of decision and push yourself to make the right decision. Don't hesitate — do it! Pretty soon the healthy choices will become habits.

+ Boost your calcium consumption with calcium-fortified juices, breads and cereals, soy products, and dark green, leafy vegetables such as collard greens and kale.

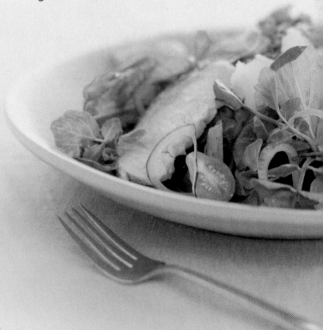

BREAK 5

No eating at restaurants

unless the meal fits the program

What:

Either don't eat out, or if you do, make sure you order foods and beverages that fit the habits in *Lose It!*

Why:

Eating out is associated with weight gain. The tantalizing sights and smells of a restaurant, deli counter, bakery display, food court or concession stand entice you with high-calorie menu items, often at times when you're not really hungry. The outcome is usually far too many calories. In addition, most — if not all — restaurants serve large portions.

HOW
↓

+ If time is an issue, find recipes for quick, easy-to-fix — and healthy — home meals. For example, serve a fresh salad with fat-free dressing, a whole-grain roll and fruit.

+ Keep on hand staple ingredients to make basic dishes at home. For example, mix together rice, beans and spices for a Tex-Mex casserole, served with your favorite salsa on the side.

+ On days when you're pressed for time, stop at a deli or grocery store on your way home and purchase a healthy sandwich, soup or prepared entrée that's low calorie and low fat.

If eating out:

+ Avoid common appetizers, which often aren't the healthiest items on the menu and tend to be a source of hidden calories. If you do have an appetizer, have vegetables, fruit or fish.

+ Because restaurant portions are large, eat slowly, and as soon as you start to feel full, put the rest of the meal into a takeout box for another meal later.

- Pick broth-based or tomato-based soups over creamed soups and chowders.

- Focus on vegetables and fruits as prominent parts of the meal.

- Request a plain vegetable salad and use low-fat dressings.

- Choose steamed vegetables, baked potato, boiled new potatoes, brown or wild rice, or fresh fruit instead of french fries, potato chips or mayonnaise-based salads such as potato salad.

- Skip dessert. If you just can't resist, have fresh fruit for dessert.

- Identify restaurants that specialize in healthy meals. If you're traveling, ask hotel attendants for suggestions.

- Don't hesitate to make special requests. Most restaurants will honor them.

- Make plans for the entire day if you know you're going out to eat. For example, have a lighter lunch if you're eating supper at a restaurant. You can also schedule extra exercise time.

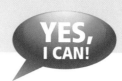

YES, I CAN!

Be prepared for challenges in a variety of situations. Use your problem-solving skills to come up with solutions that work best for you. But don't include "giving up" as one of your solutions!

- Try not to skip meals before you eat out. You may arrive at the restaurant famished and be tempted to eat too much and too fast. Have a light, healthy snack before you go out to blunt your hunger.

- Watch out for calorie-laden "extras," such as the pre-dinner breadbasket or chip bowl, that often accompany a meal.

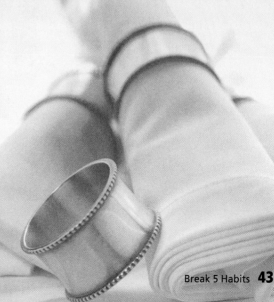

Chapter 4
Adopt
5 Bonus Habits

The Add 5 Habits and Break 5 Habits in *Lose It!* are must-dos. The 5 Bonus Habits here are optional but recommended. They're all associated with weight loss. The more of them you follow — and the more closely you follow them — the more successful you're likely to be in your weight-loss efforts.

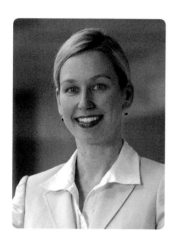

**Kristin Vickers
Douglas, Ph.D.**
Psychiatry & Psychology

The bonus habits in this chapter include keeping records of your activity and eating, and writing down your health goals. Although research tells us that this is effective, I'll be honest with you — many people don't like this at first. Some look at their eating and exercise records and feel frustrated or disappointed. Others initially think that recording goals and health behaviors is busywork, and they find it a real hassle.

The goal of recording what you plan to do (your goal), and what you really do (eating and exercise records) is to find out what's working for you and discover opportunities for change. It's detective work, really. You look for patterns and problems and then get creative about how to refine your plan for better results.

There's no reason to be self-critical and ashamed when things don't go your way. Setbacks and unmet goals are opportunities to learn. You can modify your goals, and the steps to reach those goals, so that they are realistic and relevant. Approach your records with curiosity rather than negativity: I wonder what will work best for increasing exercise, my goal from last week or my goal from this week? I wonder if I do end up eating more on days that I skip breakfast?

As you learn more about what works for you, and as you start seeing progress with your goals and eating and exercise records, you'll have even more motivation to set goals that both challenge you and fit realistically with your unique life.

BONUS 1

Keep food records

write down everything you eat

What:

Keep a record of everything you eat and drink throughout the day, including types of food and the amounts. **JOT IT ▸**

Why:

Record keeping lets you know exactly what and how much you're eating. It also allows you to identify problem patterns in your eating behavior. People who keep food records are more successful at weight loss.

HOW ↓

✦ Use *The Mayo Clinic Diet Journal* or a notebook to write down *everything* you eat. And *everything* means *everything*. **JOT IT ▸**

✦ You may need to estimate amounts in different measures. For fresh vegetables or fruits, note the size (small, medium or large). For pasta, rice, soups and beverages, indicate the number of cups or spoons.

For baked goods, use approximate dimensions. For meat, poultry and fish, use approximate weight or size. See pages 208-235 for common pyramid food group serving sizes.

✦ For mixed entrees such as casseroles, try to list the main ingredients.

✦ Pay attention to spreads, gravies and condiments that may accompany a food item. Accompaniments may have the most calories of anything you eat.

✦ If known, include the method of preparation, such as fried, baked or broiled.

✦ Don't forget to record snacks and other small items. They can add up!

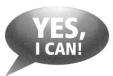
+ Write down all beverages you drink, including types (water, milk, juice) and how much you drink.

+ Keep your journal with you at all times so you can write down what you've eaten right away and don't have to try to remember later.

If you're unhappy with how your weight makes you look, take a photo of yourself, keep it with you at all times, and look at it when you're facing a challenge. Tell yourself, "I'm making progress and I'm not going back!"

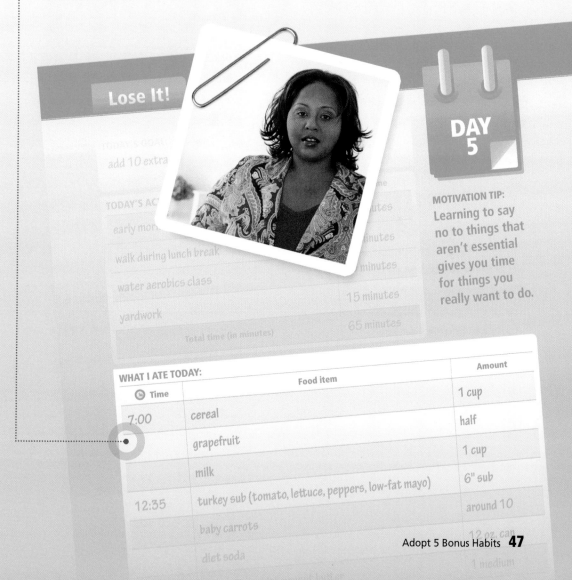

Lose It!

TODAY'S GOAL
add 10 extra

TODAY'S ACTIVITY
early morning
walk during lunch break
water aerobics class
yardwork

Total time (in minutes)

... minutes
... minutes
... minutes
15 minutes
65 minutes

DAY 5

MOTIVATION TIP:
Learning to say no to things that aren't essential gives you time for things you really want to do.

WHAT I ATE TODAY:

🕐 Time	Food item	Amount
7:00	cereal	1 cup
	grapefruit	half
	milk	1 cup
12:35	turkey sub (tomato, lettuce, peppers, low-fat mayo)	6" sub
	baby carrots	around 10
	diet soda	12 oz. can
		1 medium

BONUS 2

Keep activity records

type of activity, duration and intensity

What:

Record all your exercise and physical activity throughout the day, including the type and duration. JOT IT ▶

Why:

Record keeping helps you track the variety of activities and exercises that make up your day. Keeping a daily activity record for at least two weeks helps you to be accountable and should help you establish a regular exercise routine. Seeing your progress can build confidence and inspire you to set higher goals.

+ List on your journal activity record all household chores, hobbies, recreational activities and exercise you do. Indicate the total amount of time for each activity. Enter only those activities that last five minutes or longer. **JOT IT ▶**

+ Be aware of how intense an activity feels to you at the time you're doing it. Indicators are your heart rate, your breathing rate, perspiration and muscle fatigue. Take note of how slow or fast you performed each activity.

+ If you're walking or jogging, estimate the approximate distance you covered or the time you spent doing the activity. You may find it helpful to carry a watch or pedometer for this purpose.

+ You may wish to include in your journal other information, such as weather conditions, type of terrain, and joint or muscle aches, that you feel is important to your program.

+ Don't become an overachiever because you feel pressure to fill up your activity record. The record should reflect reasonable (and achievable) exercise goals that you've set for yourself — and not make you a workout warrior. Do what's safe and comfortable, even if that may mean leaving a few blank lines in your record.

+ Any activity you do is good, but the most benefit for you in terms of weight loss comes from moderately intense activity. See pages 90-97 and 172-179 for more details on calorie-burning activities. These include brisk walking at 3 to 4 miles per hour, swimming laps, bicycling, raking leaves and washing your car.

+ Use the information that you've written in your activity record to help you plan to make exercise and other physical activities an important part of your regular daily schedule.

YES, I CAN!

Look at this program as a game — each day is a contest, and you chalk up a win if you do most of the habits on a day (and a loss if you don't). Shoot for a "winning season" over the two weeks of *Lose It!* Go for 14-0!

Lose It!

DAILY RECORD · DAY 5

RD · DAY 6

TODAY'S GOAL:
add 10 extra minutes of exercise to my walking routine!

DAY 5

TODAY'S ACTIVITIES:	🕐 Time
early morning walk	10 minutes
walk during lunch break	10 minutes
water aerobics class	30 minutes
yardwork	15 minutes

MOTIVATION TIP:
Learning to say no to things that aren't essential gives you time for things you

BONUS 3

Move more!

walk or exercise for 60 minutes or more every day

HOW

What:

Increase your walking or exercise to 60 minutes or more every day. This doesn't have to be 60 minutes in addition to the 30 minutes or more in the earlier habit, Move! It's 60 minutes or more total. Of course, the more the better, within reason.

Why:

Increasing your physical activity to at least 60 minutes each day burns more calories and increases the health benefits you receive.

+ In this order, increase the frequency, duration and intensity of your walking or exercise. The table on page 174 shows how to gradually increase the frequency and duration of a walking program. There are several ways to vary walking intensity, for example, by lengthening your stride, swinging your arms more, increasing your speed or walking up hills.

+ If you've been inactive for a while, be cautious with a 60-minute workout. Be sure to warm up and start slowly. Initially, it's enough that you're doing something daily. Your health and safety are the highest priority.

+ Keep the intensity low enough that you can quickly build up to 30 minutes throughout the day or at a time. Once you're comfortable with a longer duration, increase the intensity. Eventually try to increase to 60 minutes or more a day, and then once again increase the intensity of your activity.

- Take into account medical or physical limitations in determining what's appropriate for you to do, but don't let lack of time or resistance to change be an excuse for not walking or exercising.

- Put walking or exercise on your schedule, much as you would any important appointment, and don't cancel it for something else. You're more likely to do it if you schedule it. It's one of the most important things you can do in your day.

- With a pedometer, record how many steps you take each day for three consecutive days. Add the daily totals and divide by three to calculate your average number of steps each day. Set a goal to increase this average by either 2,000 or 3,000 steps a day until you reach a total of 10,000 daily steps. **JOT IT** ▶

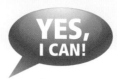

Look for excuses to exercise rather than excuses not to exercise. Get past the first five or 10 minutes and the rest is easy, and the more frequently you exercise, the more you'll want to exercise.

- To prevent boredom, consider doing a variety of activities rather than just one. For example, rotate between walking, bicycling and swimming, with a dance or aerobics class thrown in as well. Or change your routine, such as switching between early morning and late afternoon exercise times. Work out with a friend or a group.

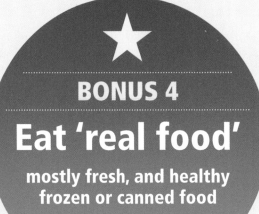

BONUS 4

Eat 'real food'

mostly fresh, and healthy frozen or canned food

What:

Eat only food that's in its natural state or is lightly processed — "real food." Limit or avoid more-processed foods, such as many canned and most boxed and convenience foods.

Why:

Food is processed to make it safe, available and convenient to use, but the processing may add unwanted fat, sugar, calories and salt. "Real food" is loaded with vitamins, minerals, fiber, antioxidants and other nutrients. Fast food is often filled with empty calories. Not everything that's processed is bad — but it's up to you to make the healthiest choices. "Real food" is often grown more locally and doesn't have as much packaging.

HOW

+ You can prepare a healthy meal almost as quickly as you can using highly processed convenience foods. The key is planning ahead so that you have on hand all the ingredients you'll need.

+ Start planning your menus with plenty of fresh fruits and vegetables. Then add whole-grain carbohydrates — brown rice and whole-grain pastas as sides or as a base for the main meal.

+ Use lean sources of protein — fish, chicken, meat, tofu — in amounts no larger than a deck of cards. Prepare them in a manner that won't add a lot of fat and calories to your diet.

+ Whole foods have been minimally processed or changed from their natural state and retain most of their nutrients. Often, you'll find whole foods, such as fresh vegetables, fruits, fish and meat, on the outside aisles of a supermarket.

+ Freezing preserves the nutrients in vegetables and fruits, although the process may change their appearance slightly. Frozen vegetables and fruits can be quickly thawed under running water and added to salads or other dishes.

- If you do use prepared food products, read the Nutrition Facts food labels on the package. Choose ones with fewer calories. In general, the least processed ones have the shortest list of ingredients.

- Rinse canned vegetables, beans and legumes in water to remove some of the excess sodium added during processing.

- Keep a stockpile of simple menu ideas in reserve that include common ingredients and require 20 minutes or less to prepare. These recipes come in handy on days when plans change or you're feeling rushed or uninspired.

- Many groceries stock a variety of fresh vegetables and fruits that are packaged and ready for immediate use out of the bag. The stores may also package lean meats that have been trimmed and pre-cut for dishes such as stir-fries or kebabs.

- Look for ways to ease the stress of meal preparation. For example, slice and chop fresh ingredients the evening before, and then refrigerate them in a sealed container overnight. In the same way, dry ingredients can be mixed together on the day before.

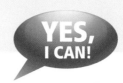

YES, I CAN!

Picture yourself doing something that you've always wanted to do but which your weight has prevented. Bring that image to mind throughout the day, especially when faced with a challenge.

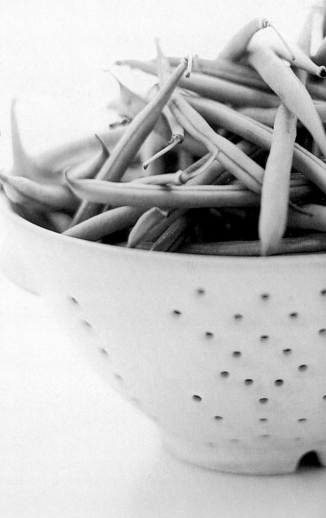

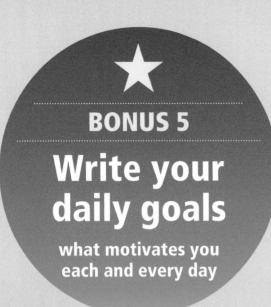

BONUS 5

Write your daily goals

what motivates you each and every day

What:

Every day write down a goal that you can take action on and achieve during that day. **JOT IT** ▶

Why:

Your overall weight goal can often be met through a series of smaller performance goals that build on each other. Goal setting keeps you motivated and helps you stick with your program.

HOW
↓

✦ Before you go to bed, write down a goal or inspirational message and tape it to the wall next to your bed so it's the first thing you see in the morning. Examples of goals might be eating at least four vegetable servings, not eating at bedtime, walking an extra three minutes or climbing an extra set of stairs (instead of using the elevator).

✦ Put your written goal where you can see it throughout the day. Read it several times a day to keep yourself motivated.

✦ Avoid daily goals based on weight loss, as your weight may vary from day to day due to fluid fluctuations in your body. When you achieve goals in activity and diet, weight loss should follow.

✦ Cast your goals in a positive light. Avoid resolute commands using "should," "must," "can't" or "won't." You subconsciously pick up on the negativity, which can lead to quick discouragement and failure. For example, rather than saying, "I won't eat any more junk food for snacks," offer a solution such as, "I'll have a piece of fruit ready when I'm hungry between meals."

- Make sure your goals are *your* goals and not someone else's.

- Be sure to give yourself a pat on the back when you reach a goal. Rewards are an important part of the process, whether it's a simple foot massage or just time to relax.

- If you get discouraged, review your goals for ways in which you've succeeded in changing your eating and exercise habits. Remember that your efforts will likely have health benefits you may not even realize.

- Write your goals for today, not for to-morrow. Just as in many aspects of life, when a goal is set for the future, it's eas-ier for you to put it off — and it remains "for tomorrow." Rather than, "I need to start walking more," write, "Today, I'm walking an extra 10 minutes."

- Setting a realistic goal doesn't mean it's an easy goal. It's true that there's danger in setting the bar too high. Nevertheless, you can judge a goal based on how it challenges your skills and resources — it should stretch them a little — and how

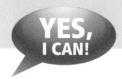

YES, I CAN!

Focus on today, not yesterday or tomorrow. Take it one day at a time, and your efforts will add up to success.

committed you need to be — it should require some effort.

- You may find yourself having to rephrase or rewrite a goal after you've tried it for a while. That's not a problem if you're fine-tuning the goal to meet different circumstances or you find the goal too challenging. It's not OK if you're chang-ing the goal simply out of convenience.

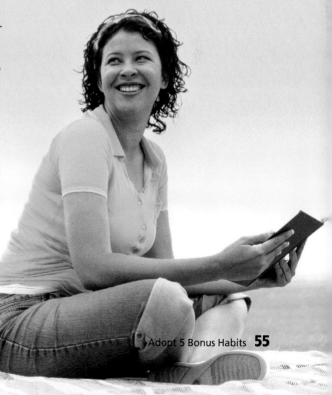

Chapter 5
What have you learned?

You're two weeks into a lifetime of better eating, moving more and enjoying a healthier weight. But it's time to see what you can learn from what you've already done, so you can be even more successful in the future.

Congratulations! You've just completed *Lose It!*, the first two weeks of *The Mayo Clinic Diet.* Now it's time for reflection. It's time to see how you did and to figure out what you can learn from *Lose It!* that will help you be successful in the *Live It!* phase of the diet.

As you analyze your *Lose It!* results, pat yourself on the back if you did well, but don't be too hard on yourself if you weren't perfect.

The habits in *Lose It!* are "stretch goals." They're designed to bump you out of your comfort zone in a rather dramatic way and head you in a different direction. (And remember, your comfort zone is probably what got you where you don't want to be with your weight in the first place.)

Odds are, even if you aced these first two weeks, you won't be able to maintain all 15 habits long term — at least to the degree asked for in *Lose It!* But that's OK. You're after the patterns rather than perfection — overall, eat more vegetables and fruits than other foods; in general, move more (a lot more). You get the picture.

Looking forward

In the weeks ahead, occasionally take time to reconfirm your commitment to weight control. Review your reasons for wanting a healthy weight and the benefits of a healthier lifestyle.

Consider factors that interfere with your success, and look for solutions. Over time, you may need to adapt your plan to changing circumstances.

Hopefully in *Lose It!*, you've learned a few habits that will help you be successful in *Live It!*, and you've found a direction you can maintain long term.

While you're evaluating your *Lose It!* results, don't rest on your laurels — you need to plow ahead into *Live It!* There's no break between the two phases of the diet. Take what you learned from *Lose It!* and translate it into your personal plan for success in *Live It!*

Strictly following the *Lose It!* habits is just for two weeks, but your goal is to establish a general direction that you can more loosely maintain — yet still benefit from — in *Live It!* (and forever).

Analyzing your results

Lose It! is all about habits — changing old ones that contributed to your weight gain and adopting new ones that help you lose weight.

Analyzing your results from the two weeks of *Lose It!* can give you an idea of what's most effective in helping you establish or break these habits.

Note the emphasis on *you*. What works for someone else might not work for you, and vice versa.

By analyzing the Habit Tracker, Daily Goals, and food and activity records you kept during *Lose It!*, you can identify personal strategies, patterns and motivators to carry over and build on in the *Live It!* phase of the diet. This review will also help if you decide to repeat *Lose It!*

To analyze your *Lose It!* results, use the following steps as a guide. You can use the *Lose It!* review form in *The Mayo Clinic Diet Journal* **JOT IT ▶** to record your results, or you can use a notebook. Here we go:

1 Using your Habit Tracker, add across the number of days you followed each habit. Do each week individually, then combine the totals for the two weeks. See the example on the next page.

+ Which habits were strengths for you?

+ List several reasons why you did well on those habits.

+ Which habits did you not follow as well?

+ List several reasons why these habits were more challenging.

+ For each reason why these habits were challenging, think of a couple of strategies for doing better. Use chapters 14 (pages 132-141) and 15 (pages 142-155) and the Action Guide (pages 180-207) for help. Come up with at least one strategy you can use right away when you encounter a challenging situation. Write down your ideas.

Habit Tracker

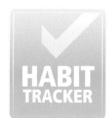

✔ Check if done

	Day 1	Day 2	Day 3	Day 4	Day 5	Day 6	Day 7	TOTALS
ADD 5 HABITS								
1. Eat a healthy breakfast	✔	✔		✔		✔	✔	5
2. Eat vegetables and fruits	✔	✔	✔		✔		✔	5
3. Eat whole grains	✔	✔	✔	✔		✔	✔	6
4. Eat healthy fats	✔	✔	✔	✔	✔		✔	6
5. Move!	✔		✔		✔	✔	✔	5
BREAK 5 HABITS								
1. No TV while eating			✔		✔		✔	3
2. No sugar	✔	✔	✔		✔	✔	✔	6
3. No snacks	✔	✔	✔	✔		✔	✔	6
4. Only moderate meat and dairy	✔	✔	✔	✔	✔		✔	6
5. No eating at restaurants	✔	✔	✔	✔	✔			6
5 BONUS HABITS								
1. Keep diet records	✔	✔	✔	✔	✔	✔	✔	7
2. Keep exercise/activity records	✔	✔	✔	✔	✔	✔	✔	7
3. Move more!	✔						✔	2
4. Eat "real" food	✔	✔		✔			✔	4
5. Write your daily goals	✔	✔	✔	✔	✔	✔	✔	7
TOTALS:	**14**	**12**	**12**	**10**	**10**	**9**	**14**	

2 Using your Habit Tracker, add down each column to total the number of habits you followed each day. **JOT IT** ▸

+ Which days of the week did you do better?

+ List reasons why you did better on those days. Look at your daily journal and Daily Goals to pick up clues.

+ On which days did you not follow the habits as well?

+ List reasons why it was more challenging on those days. Use your daily journal and Daily Goals to look for clues. Also look at your Habit Tracker to identify possible patterns: Did you do better at the beginning of the week but lose momentum by the end of the week? Is there a particular day of the week that poses special challenges?

+ For each reason why it was more challenging on certain days, think of a few strategies for doing better. Use chapters 14 (pages 132-141) and

15 (pages 142-155) and the Action Guide (pages 180-207) for help. Come up with at least one strategy you can implement right away when you encounter a challenging situation. Write down your ideas.

3 Look at the Yes, I Can! **YES, I CAN!** motivation messages associated with each habit. Rank each one on a 1 to 5 scale, with 1 being not helpful and 5 being very helpful. Note those that were most helpful.

4 For your Daily Goals, do the same analysis as in 3 above.

5 Total your weight loss recorded on days 7 and 14 and enter on the *Lose It!* review page.

+ Did you lose more weight in one week than in the other? If so, consider factors from numbers 1 to 4 above that may have played a role. Write these down.

What worked and what didn't

Now that you've done the math, look back over your assessment and identify what worked and what didn't. Use a highlighter to mark those things that will be helpful, so they'll be easy to flip back to.

As you analyze your assessment, consider questions such as these, and possible solutions:

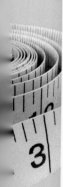

+ What were my top problem areas?

+ Do I encounter challenges in certain places — the office, at home, at the mall — or on certain days?

+ Are there "people issues" (lack of support) that I need to address?

+ How do I best handle overcoming challenges, and how can I use that information in brainstorming solutions for challenges?

Use chapters 14 and 15 and the Action Guide for ideas, but remember that this is about you — when you come up with your own solutions, you're more likely to be successful.

As you transition into *Live It!*, perhaps your biggest challenge will be keeping yourself from sliding back into old habits. As you go through *Live It!*, occasionally revisit the pages of *Lose It!* and your assessment, to help keep yourself on track.

Now, on to *Live It!*

Part 2 *Live It!*

Lose It! gave you a quick start. *Live It!* puts you on a path you can enjoy for a lifetime.

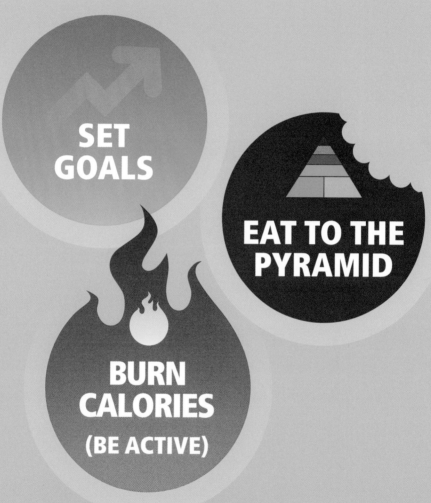

SET GOALS

EAT TO THE PYRAMID

BURN CALORIES (BE ACTIVE)

A healthy, effective, common-sense approach to weight loss

Chapter 6
Preparing to *Live It!*

Lose It! is like the "grab-'em-by-an-arm-and-a-leg-and-throw-'em-in" method of learning to swim — not very subtle or refined, but the results are immediate. Now that you know how to dog paddle, *Live It!* gives you the tools and techniques to help you swim the distance in your quest for a healthy weight.

If you're doing this right, you're reading this chapter while you're still in (or before you even start) *Lose It!* You need to read ahead so you're prepared for what's to come and don't miss a beat. There's no break between *Lose It!* and *Live It!* No rest for the weary.

Lose It! is designed to build momentum. Don't let that slow now. Take the *Lose It!* habits and keep applying them in a general way in *Live It!* You may not want — or be able — to follow all of them to the degree you did in *Lose It!*, but keep the general principles in play.

In *Live It!* you'll:

+ Set weight-loss goals.

+ Learn a pattern of eating that will help you meet those goals.

+ Acquire the ability to determine at a glance the number of calories in food (well, not the exact number of calories, but a close-enough measurement — servings).

+ Find ways to speed the process by burning more calories.

Make it a habit!

Here's all it takes to enjoy a lifetime with *Live It!*

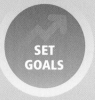

SET GOALS

Set daily goals for food servings and longer term weight goals.

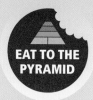

EAT TO THE PYRAMID

Make informed food choices by eating to the Mayo Clinic Healthy Weight Pyramid.

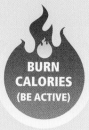

BURN CALORIES (BE ACTIVE)

Be more active to burn more calories (and improve your health).

Setting your weight-loss goal

How much do you want to weigh? Less than you do now, or you wouldn't be reading this. You may have a number in mind — something more concrete than "less." But before you zero in on a weight-loss goal, let's talk a bit about goals. It may make a difference in how well you succeed.

Two types of goals

Two types of goals can help or hurt your weight-loss effort:

+ **Outcome goals.** An outcome goal focuses on an end result. "I want to weigh 125 pounds," or "I want to lose 30 pounds."

+ **Performance goals.** A performance goal focuses on a process or action. "I will walk 30 minutes each day," or "I will eat four servings of vegetables each day."

Performance goals can help you achieve outcome goals. Setting an outcome goal without performance

Be SMART about goals

All goals — outcome and performance goals, and long-term and intermediate goals — should be:

+ **Specific** — State exactly what you want to achieve, how you're going to do it and when you want to achieve it.
+ **Measurable** — How will you know if you've reached your goal if you can't measure it?
+ **Attainable** — Set a goal that you have sufficient time and resources to achieve.
+ **Realistic** — Set a goal that is within your capabilities. If you've never been remotely close to a size 4, is that realistic? If your goal is not realistic, you'll get discouraged (and discouragement can lead to binge eating, and you know where that leads).
+ **Trackable** — Tracking your progress keeps you motivated. Jot down your results in *The Mayo Clinic Diet Journal* or a notebook. **JOT IT** ▶

goals is like trying to run a marathon without training for it — you don't have much chance for success (and it's likely to be a painful experience). An outcome goal becomes easier to achieve when it's coupled with performance goals that provide the steps necessary to get you to the desired outcome.

For weight loss, you don't necessarily even need an outcome goal. Some people find that just focusing on the process of losing weight (using performance goals) is more effective, and their weight eventually hits a satisfying level. Others find that aiming for a specific target weight helps keep them motivated and on track.

Both approaches can work. Whichever you use, just be SMART about setting your goals (see page 66).

Breaking it down helps

If you're setting a specific weight-loss outcome goal, breaking your goal into steps can help keep you motivated as you focus on and achieve those intermediate goals.

If you want to lose, say, 25 pounds in three months, you could break it down to 8 pounds during the two weeks of the *Lose It!* phase, then 6 more by the end of the first month of *Live It!*, 6 more in the second month, and another 5 in the third month.

Breaking down goals is more important the more weight you want to lose. Goals far in the future are harder to attain without intermediate goals to keep you focused and motivated. And don't forget the performance goals to help you get there.

So what's your goal?

There's really no wrong answer when setting a weight-loss goal, as long as your goal weight is safe (healthy) and realistic. What might a realistic goal be? Depending on your weight, 10 percent of your current weight might be a good start. That's 18 pounds if you weigh 180 pounds, or 25 pounds if you weigh 250 (and so on).

You can take a look at the body mass index chart on page 107 for a guide to a healthy weight. That may or may not be realistic for you, and if it is, it may take several steps (intermediate goals) to get there. Your doctor may be able to help you set a specific goal based on your health.

Whether you're setting a specific goal or focusing on performance goals, write your goals down in *The Mayo Clinic Diet Journal* or in a notebook. JOT IT ▸ Use them to keep yourself motivated along the way.

Selecting your daily calorie goal

Calories-in minus calories-out equals weight gain or weight loss. Here, we're going to focus on the calories-in part.

To lose weight, you need to set a daily goal for the number of calories to consume (one of those performance-oriented goals). If you eat 500 fewer calories each day than you normally do

It's OK to dream big

Big things don't happen unless you have big aspirations. But recognize that big things typically don't happen without big efforts.

Champion athletes don't become champions and then start training like one. It's the other way around — they dream big, do the necessary planning and preparation, and then work their tails off in hopes that their training and dedication pay off.

So dream big if you want to — keeping realism in mind — but prepare (set intermediate and performance goals) for a championship effort to reach that big goal.

Your daily calorie level for healthy weight loss

Weight in pounds	Starting calorie goal			
Women	**1,200**	**1,400**	**1,600**	**1,800**
250 or less	✔			
251 to 300		✔		
301 or more			✔	
Men	**1,200**	**1,400**	**1,600**	**1,800**
250 or less		✔		
251 to 300			✔	
301 or more				✔

and keep your activity level the same, you'll lose about 1 pound in a week. That's because 3,500 calories equals about a pound of body fat.

In *Live It!*, the goal is to lose about 1 to 2 pounds a week, so that means consuming at least 500 to 1,000 calories a day less than you normally do. (Keep in mind that you can help this equation by burning more calories, but we'll get to that later.)

You can go through the process of tracking your calorie intake for several days, averaging it and then subtracting 500 to 1,000 calories to get a goal, but that's a lot of work and not really necessary. Instead, we've simplified things with the accompanying table, which is based on average calorie intakes needed to result in a 1- to 2-pound-a-week weight loss. Just find your current weight and read across to the desired daily calorie level.

These are good calorie levels to start with. You can adjust them based on your own goals and how quickly you want to lose weight. If you feel exceptionally hungry or lose weight too quickly, consider moving up to the next calorie level. If you're moving down a level, don't drop below the

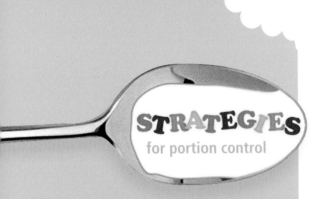

Here are strategies to help you control the portions of food you eat:

- **Eat slowly.** When you eat too fast, your brain doesn't get the signal that you're full until it's too late and you've already overeaten.
- **See what you eat.** Don't eat directly from a container. Seeing food on a plate or in a bowl gives you a better sense of portion size.
- **Focus on your food.** Watching television, reading or working while you eat distracts you. Before you know it, you've eaten more than you want to.
- **Serve smaller amounts.** Take slightly less than what you think you'll eat. Using a smaller plate or bowl makes less food seem like more.
- **Don't feel obligated to clean your plate.** Stop eating as soon as you feel satisfied. Those extra bites of food that you're trying not to waste add unneeded calories. But better yet, take smaller portions to begin with so you don't waste food.

lowest level listed. Fewer than 1,200 daily calories for women and 1,400 for men generally aren't recommended because you may not get enough nutrients.

Determining your daily servings

Now you know how many calories you want to eat in a day, but the thing is, you don't eat calories, you eat food.

You can go through some pretty detailed tracking and analysis to convert the food you eat into calories, but again, that really isn't necessary. To simplify things, this program focuses on servings from food groups in the Mayo Clinic Healthy Weight Pyramid rather than on calories.

Using your daily calorie goal, look at the accompanying table to determine the number of pyramid servings of various foods to eat. Tracking these is a lot easier than counting calories, and it gives a "close-enough" measurement of calorie intake. It also provides a guide to what kind of foods to eat, ensuring that you get a balanced diet.

Serving recommendations for daily calorie goals

Food group		Daily calorie goals				
		1,200	1,400	1,600	1,800	2,000
V	Vegetables	4 or more	4 or more	5 or more	5 or more	5 or more
F	Fruits	3 or more	4 or more	5 or more	5 or more	5 or more
C	Carbohydrates	4	5	6	7	8
PD	Protein/Dairy	3	4	5	6	7
Ft	Fats	3	3	3	4	5

Don't freak when you see you'll be eating at least four servings of vegetables a day and three servings of fruit. As you'll see in the following pages, what you think of as a serving may not be all that much. And, we'll give you plenty of tips along the way to help you meet your servings goals.

A portion is not necessarily a serving

"I can't do that!" might have been your first reaction to seeing how many servings of some foods you'll be eating in *The Mayo Clinic Diet.*

But hold on — you may be confusing servings with portions.

With the Mayo Clinic Healthy Weight Pyramid, a serving is an exact amount of food, defined by common measurements such as cups, ounces and tablespoons. Don't confuse that with a portion, which is the amount of food you put on your plate. A portion of food may contain several servings.

Serving sizes vary from one pyramid food group to the next, due to variation in their calorie content. For example, a pyramid serving of vegetables has around 25 calories, while a pyramid serving of carbohydrates has around 70 calories.

But you don't need to memorize a full inventory of food serving sizes or carry measuring cups with you to meals. As the table on the next page shows, you can use common visual cues to estimate servings. And in Chapter 8 (pages 80-89), we'll walk you through how to analyze complete meals — breakfast, lunch and dinner — for *close-enough* estimates of servings.

Serving sizes at a glance

The following page provides some visual cues to help you gauge Mayo Clinic Healthy Weight Pyramid serving sizes of various foods. Use it and the information in Chapter 8 to track your daily servings.

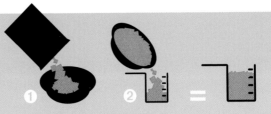

Making sense of servings

Estimating your servings at meals is a great way to control the calories you consume. Unfortunately, the eye can be deceiving. Most people habitually, and unintentionally, underestimate the number of servings they eat. This means they consume more calories than they think they're getting, and they can't understand why they're gaining weight. Here's an exercise to help you get a better sense of servings.

Pour dry cereal into a bowl until you have what you think is about ½ cup. Don't use a measuring device, just depend on your own estimation.

Now pour the cereal out of the bowl and into a measuring cup. How close did you come to ½ cup? If you overestimated, don't feel discouraged. Most people imagine ½ cup being a greater amount than it actually is. Try this exercise a few more times to see if you can get a closer estimate. One serving of dry cereal is the equivalent of ½ cup.

You can try this same exercise the next time you're cooking pasta. After you've drained the cooked pasta, try putting approximately ½ cup into a bowl, then put it into a measuring cup. One serving of cooked pasta is about ½ cup.

Try this exercise with favorite foods that you frequently eat. The more you practice, the more control you'll have over portion sizes when you're getting ready for meals.

Quick guide to serving sizes

Vegetables	Calories	Visual cue
1 cup broccoli	25	1 baseball
2 cups raw, leafy greens	25	2 baseballs

Fruits	Calories	Visual cue
½ cup sliced fruit	60	Tennis ball
1 small apple or medium orange	60	Tennis ball

Carbohydrates	Calories	Visual cue
½ cup pasta or dried cereal	70	Hockey puck
½ bagel	70	Hockey puck
1 slice whole-grain bread	70	Hockey puck
½ medium baked potato	70	Hockey puck

Protein/Dairy	Calories	Visual cue
3 ounces of fish	110	Deck of cards
2-2½ ounces of meat	110	⅔ deck of cards
1½-2 ounces of hard cheese	110	⅓ deck of cards

Fats	Calories	Visual cue
1½ teaspoons peanut butter	45	2 dice
1 teaspoon butter or margarine	45	1 die

These visual cues can help you use the food lists on pages 208 to 235.

EAT TO THE PYRAMID

Chapter 7
Eating to the Pyramid

Eating is one of life's great pleasures. Eating well and losing weight *can* go hand in hand. This chapter shows you how.

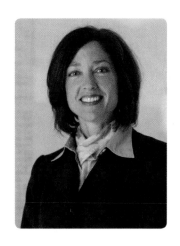

Rose Prissel, R.D.
Clinical Nutrition

When did it become so hard to figure out what to eat, or when to eat, or even how to eat? What happened to our ability to play?

It doesn't have to be that difficult. To enjoy eating to its fullest, keep it simple.

You probably know it's a good idea to eat your fruits and vegetables, but are you aware that you can *flavor* your food with an abundant variety of fruits or vegetables? Have you explored the tantalizing possibilities of herbs and spices?

The kitchen is one of the few places you can feel free to experiment and play with flavor combinations. You're the only judge: "Do I like it?" Discover and expand your palate every chance you get. Explore new food with a friend. Keep the excitement. Who doesn't enjoy playing?

When was the last time you fully enjoyed the experience of eating? Eat with your eyes, bringing color to your plate with fruits and vegetables. Taste with your sense of smell, creating tantalizing aromas with garlic, cinnamon or basil. Savor the coolness, heat, sharpness, the sweet, salty or sour, the smooth, coarse, chewy or crunchy.

When you enjoy something, a little goes a long way.

OK, you've got your number of servings (figured in Chapter 6). Now what do you do with them? Grab an apple to munch on, and we'll walk you through eating to the pyramid.

Eating to the pyramid is pretty simple. The pyramid's shape gives you a general direction of eating (page 18). Focus on vegetables and fruits, followed by progressively lesser amounts of whole grains, lean protein and dairy, healthy fats, and sweets.

The number of servings you figured out in Chapter 6 are your targets for each of the pyramid food groups (that apple you're eating counts as a fruit serving, so chalk one up in that category. Easy, huh?). The servings also ensure that you're getting a nutritionally balanced diet. For details on the pyramid food groups, see Chapter 13 (pages 122-131).

But unless you're going to eat only single servings of single-ingredient foods — for example, that one apple, or half a cup of pasta with no sauce — it's a little more complex (but not much) when planning what to eat for an entire day or a week. That takes a little menu planning. Here's how you do that (see example on the next page as you read on):

+ Start with a blank copy of a menu planner from *The Mayo Clinic Diet Journal.* **JOT IT** ▸ Have your daily servings goals handy.

+ Because vegetables and fruits form the foundation of the pyramid, as you plan each meal start with those first. Remember that the servings goals for vegetables and fruits are minimums, not maximums. You can consume unlimited servings of vegetables and fruits. Look for ways to serve them whole and fresh and in combination with other foods.

+ Using the food lists on pages 208-235, begin by planning breakfast (remember the first Add Habit from *Lose It!*). Want a banana? Pencil it in and check off one fruit serving. Half a bagel with a little jam? Jot them down and check off one carbohydrate and tally the sweets calories (unless it's a sugar-free jam). And so on.

MAIN MEAL OR MEALS OF THE DAY	HOW MUCH
Breakfast	
whole-grain bagel	1/2 bagel
strawberry jam	1 tbsp
banana	1 small
coffee	1 cup
Lunch	
ham sandwich	6" sub
baby carrots	1/2 cup
ranch dressing	2 tbsp
apple	1 small
water	1 cup
Dinner	
grilled chicken breast	2 1/2 oz
baby potatoes	3
steamed broccoli	2 cups
margarine	1 tsp
pear	

PYRAMID SERVINGS FOR THIS MEAL

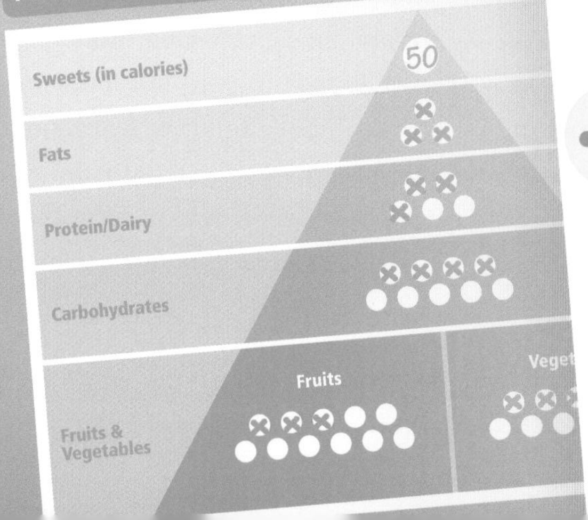

Sweets (in calories)	50
Fats	✕✕
Protein/Dairy	✕✕
Carbohydrates	●●●●●
Fruits & Vegetables	Fruits ●●●●● Veget. ✕✕ ●●●

Carbohydrates

Item (70 calories per serving)	One serving is
Animal crackers	6 crackers
Bagel, cinnamon-raisin	½ bagel (3-inch)
★ Bagel, whole-grain	½ bagel (3-inch)
★ Barley, cooked	⅓ cup
Biscuits, plain or buttermilk, from dry mix	1 small
Bread, white or sourdough	1 slice
★ Bread, whole-grain	1 slice
★ Bread, whole-wheat white	1 slice

Sweets

Item (75 calories per serving)	One serving is
Chocolate chips, semisweet	4 tablespoons
Cranberry sauce, canned, sweetened	3 tablespoons
Frosting, chocolate, ready-to-eat	1 tablespoon
Fruit butter, apple	2½ tablespoons
Gelatin dessert	½ cup
Hard candy (butterscotch, lemon drops, peppermint)	4 pieces
Honey	1 tablespoon
Jellies, jams and preserves (all varieties)	1½ tablespoons
Jellies, jams and preserves, reduced-sugar	4 tablespoons
Jelly beans	20 small or 8 large
Molasses	1½ tablespoons
Rhubarb, cooked and sweetened	¼ cup
Sugar, brown (unpacked)	2 tablespoons
Sugar, granulated, white	4 teaspoons

A c
so
wh
ch
b
m
e

Fruits

Item (60 calories per serving)	One serving is
★ Apple	1 small
Apple, dried	⅓ cup
Applesauce, sweetened	⅓ cup
★ Applesauce, unsweetened	½ cup
★ Apricot	4 whole or 8 dried halves
★ Banana	1 small
★ Berries, mixed	¾ cup
★ Blackberries	1 cup
★ Blueberries	¾ cup
★ Breadfruit	¼ cup
★ Cantaloupe (muskmelon)	1 cup cubed or ⅓ small melon
★ Cherries	15 fruits
★ Clementine	2 small
Dates	3 fruits
★ Figs	2 small
Figs, dried	3 small
★ Grapefruit	¾ cup sections or ½ large
★ Grapes, seedless, red or green	1 cup (about 30)
	2 fruits or ½ cup

FROM T

The principle
fruit serving
Clinic Diet
dried varie
raisins and
because w
they shri
piece of c
a lot of c
is still he
recomm
listed in

+ Finish planning breakfast, then proceed to lunch and dinner. Don't forget a couple of snacks (fresh vegetables and fruits are best).

+ Don't forget to count servings for what you put on vegetables and fruits (such as the ranch dressing you've been dipping those carrots into).

+ Use the mixed foods section of the food lists for foods that have more than one ingredient.

+ If at the end of the day you find that you have planned too many servings of one pyramid group and not enough of another, go back and tweak things.

That's it. There's your menu plan for a day.

There's more detail on menu planning, plus sample menus, in Chapter 16 (pages 156-165). Chapter 8 (pages 80-89) can help you learn how to determine the number of servings in mixed-food meals. And there are recipes on pages 236-245.

In addition, the following tips can help:

+ **Plan by the week.** It's more efficient to plan menus for an entire week instead of day to day. Don't get hung up on exact servings totals. If you're off target one day, make up for it on the next. Balance things over a week. Use the menu planners in *The Mayo Clinic Diet Journal* to help you plan. **JOT IT** ▸

+ **Make pleasure a priority.** Losing weight may require you to cut back on some of your favorite foods, but don't sacrifice enjoyment. That means no severe restrictions, no extreme hunger and no unrealistic expectations. Create some new favorites — there are a lot of great foods and recipes to explore!

+ **Establish a routine.** Let the rhythm of your weekly schedule determine which evenings to spend more time preparing dinner and which evenings to fall back on a convenience food (a healthy one of course). Save time by using a slow cooker. Make dishes on the weekends and refrigerate or freeze portions for the week ahead. Schedule a regular spaghetti night or a leftovers night — based on the extra portions you made at a previous meal. Don't hesitate to repeat the same menus every few weeks.

+ **Adapt menus to the season.** Use the freshest foods available for your meals — asparagus, peas and cherries in the late spring, tomatoes, corn and peaches in late summer. Recently harvested produce is often available at local farmers markets.

+ **Don't forget convenience.**
Consider convenience foods such as a favorite frozen entrée or side dish on those days when there's little time to fix meals. Just be selective about what you choose. Read the nutrition labels. Don't choose based on calories alone. Also look for items that are low in fat and that aren't loaded with sodium.

+ **Look for shortcuts.** Simplify meal preparation and save time by purchasing pre-cut vegetables and fruits, precooked meats, shredded low-fat cheeses and packaged salads.

If you're hungry, EAT!

A cardinal rule of *The Mayo Clinic Diet* is, "If you're hungry, eat!"

Starving yourself can be counterproductive and set you up for overeating later. Plus, it's just no fun.

Because *The Mayo Clinic Diet* allows unlimited consumption of vegetables and fruits, focus on those when you're hungry. They'll fill you up without giving you a lot of calories.

Frozen or canned vegetables and fruits also come in handy. Rinse canned vegetables with water to remove excess sodium. Buy fruit that's canned in its own juice rather than in syrup.

+ **Be flexible.** Every food you eat doesn't have to be an excellent source of nutrition. It's OK to eat high-fat, high-calorie foods on occasion. The main point is to *most of the time* choose foods that promote good health. They're the ones also most likely to help you lose weight.

Chapter 8
No food scales or calculators needed

A portion of food is how much you put on your plate. A pyramid serving is a specific amount of food that equals a certain number of calories. How do you determine the number of pyramid servings in a portion of food, and in which pyramid food groups they should be counted? It doesn't take complex measurements and calculations. This visual guide will help you learn to come up with estimates that are close enough.

Visual guide to servings sizes
See larger chart on page 73.

1 Vegetable serving =
1 baseball

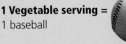

1 Fruit serving =
1 tennis ball

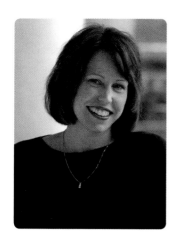

Sara Wolf, R.D.

Clinical Nutrition

A common theme that comes through loud and clear from people is that time is of the essence. "I'm busy. Please don't give me complicated eating plans. I don't have time to measure every ounce and teaspoon."

So, I say, "Then don't!"

But do learn how to estimate portion sizes and plan meals by using the tips included in this chapter — a deck of cards is the size of a serving of meat, a tennis ball is a serving of fruit, and so on. Knowing recommended portion sizes and how to combine foods in a healthy way can make meal planning and food selection a breeze.

Your ability to control portions and plan meals will make or break your weight-loss efforts. As portion and plate sizes have increased over the years, so have waistlines. To survive these trends, we must embrace different ways of eating, at home and away.

Everyone has strengths and weaknesses when it comes to portion control. Some can eat a portion-controlled, planned supper, only to graze all evening. Some never snack, but eat very large meals. And some eat all day long. Look within to find barriers to success and plan solutions that work for you.

PD Note:
The deck of cards visual cue for the Protein/ Dairy group applies only to meat servings. A deck of cards would be too much cheese and too little milk.

1 Carbohydrate serving =
1 hockey puck

1 Protein/Dairy serving =
1 deck of cards or less

1 Fat serving =
1 to 2 dice

Breakfast

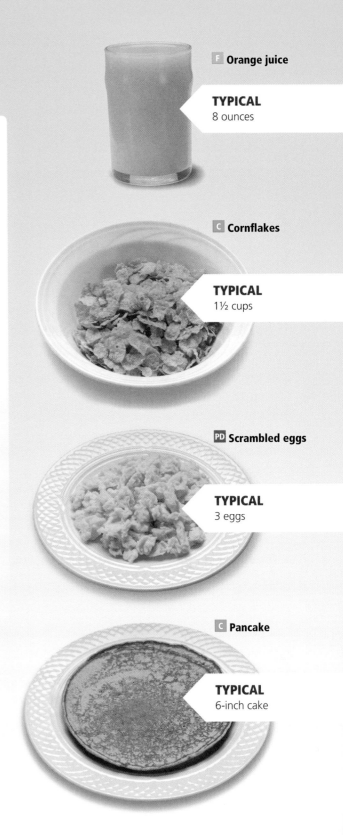

F Orange juice

TYPICAL
8 ounces

C Cornflakes

TYPICAL
1½ cups

PD Scrambled eggs

TYPICAL
3 eggs

C Pancake

TYPICAL
6-inch cake

PRACTICING PORTION CONTROL

Too often, breakfast is an all-or-nothing affair. Either it's calorie overload (eggs, bacon and hash browns) or almost no nutrition at all (coffee or soda). Breakfast should provide you with essential nutrients and give you an energy push. It should not be an occasion for thoughtless or unrestrained eating.

The challenge is to keep your breakfast portions under control. Eating too little deprives you of the important benefits of breakfast. Eating too much simply reduces the number of servings you can eat at later meals in the day.

Typical breakfast portions

Item		Food group	Servings
F	Orange juice	Fruits	2
C	Cornflakes	Carbohydrates	3
PD	Scrambled eggs	Protein/Dairy	3
C	Pancake	Carbohydrates	1½

Tip

Rule to remember!
If you control portion size, the calories tend to take care of themselves.

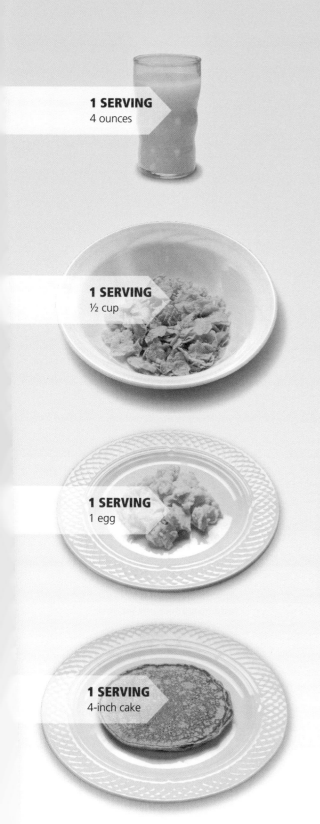

1 SERVING
4 ounces

1 SERVING
½ cup

1 SERVING
1 egg

1 SERVING
4-inch cake

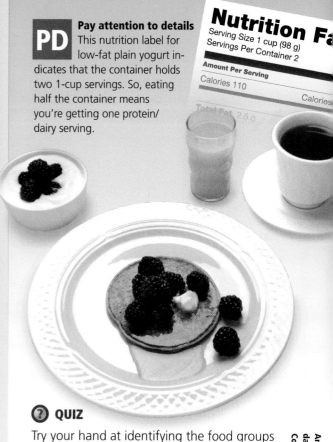

PD **Pay attention to details**
This nutrition label for low-fat plain yogurt indicates that the container holds two 1-cup servings. So, eating half the container means you're getting one protein/dairy serving.

Nutrition Fa
Serving Size 1 cup (98 g)
Servings Per Container 2

Amount Per Serving

Calories 110   Calories

Total Fat 2.5 g

? QUIZ

Try your hand at identifying the food groups in this breakfast of a pancake with trans fat-free margarine, syrup and berries, low-fat yogurt, juice and coffee. Check off the food groups and indicate the number of servings.

✔	Food group	No. of servings
☐	**V** Vegetables	
☐	**F** Fruits	
☐	**C** Carbohydrates	
☐	**PD** Protein/Dairy	
☐	**Ft** Fats	
☐	**S** Sweets	

You'll find the answer on the right-hand side of this page.

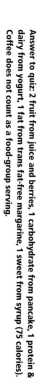

Answer to quiz: 2 fruit from juice and berries, 1 carbohydrate from pancake, 1 protein & dairy from yogurt, 1 fat from trans fat-free margarine, 1 sweet from syrup (75 calories). Coffee does not count as a food-group serving.

Lunch

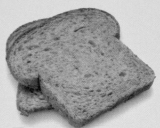

TAKING APART A SANDWICH

If you build something, you can also take it apart, right? One way to estimate servings is to mentally "take apart" the meal. That is, reverse the meal-making process until you can identify the separate ingredients. Try it on something simple, like a roast beef sandwich:

C Bread
1 slice = 1 carbohydrate serving

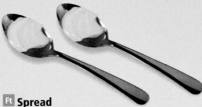

Ft Spread
2 teaspoons of mayonnaise = 1 fat serving

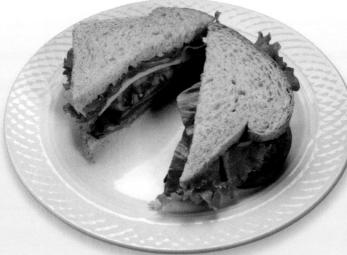

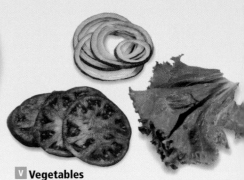

V Vegetables
Tomato slices, onion slice and lettuce = 1 vegetable serving

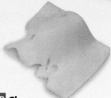

PD Cheese
2 ounces of low-fat cheese = 1 protein/dairy serving

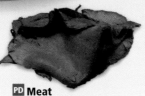

PD Meat
2 ounces of roast beef = 1 protein/dairy serving

Here's a breakdown of the food-group servings for your roast-beef sandwich:

V	Vegetables	1
F	Fruits	0
C	Carbohydrates	2
PD	Protein/Dairy	2
Ft	Fats	1
S	Sweets	0

Ft Lose the fat!
Substituting mustard for mayonnaise in your sandwich eliminates the fat serving.

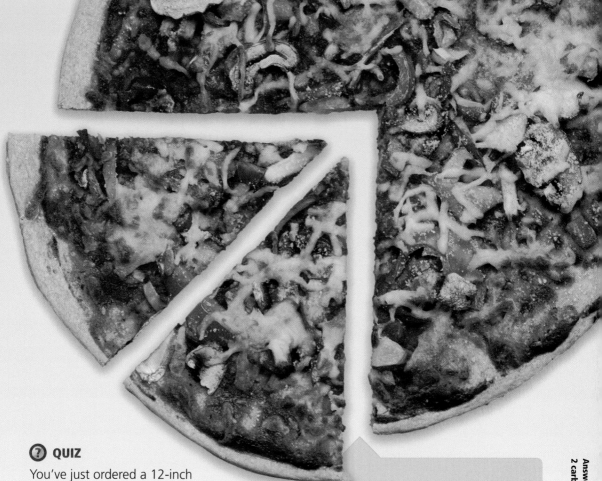

❓ QUIZ

You've just ordered a 12-inch vegetarian pizza. How many food-group servings do you think are in two slices? Put your best guess below:

✔	Food group	No. of servings
☐	**V** Vegetables	
☐	**F** Fruits	
☐	**C** Carbohydrates	
☐	**PD** Protein/Dairy	
☐	**Ft** Fats	
☐	**S** Sweets	

You'll find the answer on the right-hand side of this page.

Helpful hints to deconstruct the pizza:

+ Thin whole-wheat crust
+ Layer of tomato sauce
+ Topped with chopped onion, green pepper and mushroom
+ Sprinkled with low-fat cheese
+ "Hidden" fat used to make the pizza crust

Answer to quiz: 2 vegetable from toppings and tomato sauce, 2 carbohydrate and 2 fat from cheese and pizza crust.

Dinner

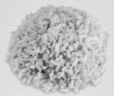

UNSCRAMBLING FOOD JUMBLES

A dish that mixes many ingredients together, such as a stir-fry, can be a special challenge for your food record. It's difficult to know how much of any single food group is a part of the delectable display of colors, shapes, textures and flavors.

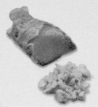

C Grain
⅓ cup cooked brown rice = 1 carbohydrate serving

V Seasonings
Chopped ginger and garlic = too little to include as a vegetable serving

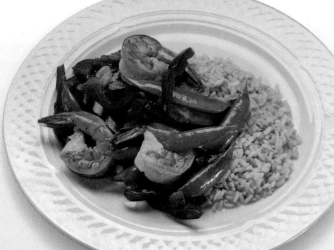

  See page 244 for this recipe

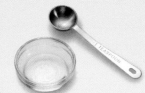

Ft Oil
1 teaspoon olive oil = 1 fat serving

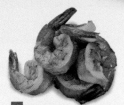

PD Meat
4 ounces shrimp (about 6 large) = 1 protein/dairy serving

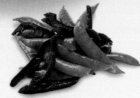

V Vegetables
1 medium bell pepper = 1 vegetable serving
¼ cup snow peas = 1 vegetable serving

Here's a breakdown of the food-group servings for the shrimp stir-fry:

V	Vegetables	2
F	Fruits	0
C	Carbohydrates	1
PD	Protein/Dairy	1
Ft	Fats	1
S	Sweets	0

Ft In general, about 1 tablespoon of oil is needed for a stir-fry, which equals 3 fat servings. However, most stir-fry recipes serve more than one person.

1 Vegetable serving =
1 baseball

1 Carbohydrate serving =
1 hockey puck

1 Protein/Dairy serving =
3 ounces of fish is
1 deck of cards

❓ QUIZ

How many servings can you estimate for this dinner of grilled salmon, Swiss chard sautéed with olive oil and garlic, and whole-wheat pasta with Parmesan cheese?

✔	Food group	No. of servings
☐	**V** Vegetables	
☐	**F** Fruits	
☐	**C** Carbohydrates	
☐	**PD** Protein/Dairy	
☐	**Ft** Fats	
☐	**S** Sweets	

You'll find the answer on the right-hand side of this page.

Pay attention to your plate

How different foods are served on your dinner plate plays a role in portion control. In general, look for portions of vegetables or fruits to take up about half the plate, and carbohydrates about one-quarter of the space. What remains is generally for protein/dairy. If you can match these proportions, you're looking at a pretty healthy meal.

Answer to quiz: 2 vegetable from Swiss chard, 2 carbohydrate from pasta, 1 protein & dairy from salmon, 2 fat from oil used to sauté Swiss chard and cheese added to pasta.

Dinner

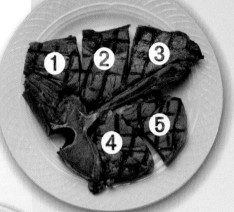

VISUAL CUES FOR SERVING SIZES

Imagine a deck of cards for a single serving of Protein/Dairy. Try it out on a grilled 20-ounce T-bone steak: Divide this amount of meat into 5 portions. Each 4-ounce piece is equal to two Protein/Dairy servings from the Mayo Clinic Healthy Weight Pyramid. Add a baked potato and tossed salad — you have a delicious dinner for the entire family.

1 Protein/Dairy serving = 2-2½ ounces of meat is ⅔ deck of cards

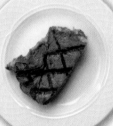

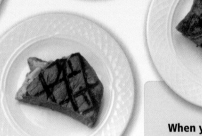

PD Chicken and turkey are low in fat, especially when the skin is removed. Fish and shellfish are even lower in fat and some varieties have omega-3 fatty acids, which are good for the heart.

When you eat beef, choose leaner cuts such as sirloin, tenderloin, round and chuck. *Lean* is defined as 8½ grams or less of total fat in 3 ounces of beef. *Extra lean* means less than 4½ grams of total fat in 3 ounces of beef.

Snacks

10 chocolate peanut candies

2 tablespoons peanuts

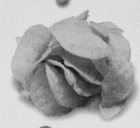

1 ounce potato chips

RECOGNIZING THE BEST OPTIONS

Different food items are pictured here in amounts equal to 100 calories. That's just about right for a snack while still allowing you to meet daily calorie goals.

You want a snack that eases hunger but doesn't dampen your appetite for regular meals. As these examples demonstrate, you can eat more of some foods than of others to reach 100 calories. That little bit more leaves you feeling fuller and may quash food cravings later on.

2 cups carrots

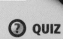

1⅔ cups grapes

3½ cups popcorn

Tip You're welcome to vary your snack choices (as long as the portions are moderate). But more often, choose snack foods that have a low energy density, such as carrots, grapes and air-popped popcorn. You can eat more of them — it's that simple.

❓ QUIZ

The Mayo Clinic Healthy Weight Pyramid recommends a daily calorie amount for sweets — 75 calories. How much of this candy bar could you eat and still be within the daily recommendation?

Regular-sized candy bars fall within a range of 220 to 280 calories a bar.

You'll find the answer on the right-hand side of this page.

Answer to quiz: Between one-third and one-fourth of this regular-size candy bar typically equals 75 calories.

Chapter 9
Burning calories

The fastest way to lose weight is to alter both sides of the equation — calories in (eating) and calories out (physical activity). This chapter will show you how to boost your weight loss by burning more calories.

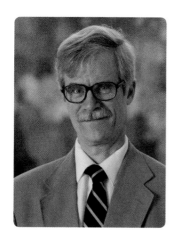

Warren Thompson, M.D.
Preventive Medicine

Our ancestors ate more than we do, yet they weighed less. Why? They were always on the move.

The television, the automobile, appliances and the changing nature of our work (switching from farming to desk jobs) have resulted in a dramatic drop in calories burned over the last 100 years. But if you increase your energy expenditure, you'll not only improve your chances of losing weight, but you'll also reduce your risk of heart disease, dementia and diabetes, and you'll feel better.

To keep weight off, increasing activity is essential. Studies show that people who lose over 30 pounds and keep it off for five years exercise (mostly by walking) an hour each day. That's a lot (but it's why our ancestors were thinner), and it's not easy. A study of highly motivated women showed that only 25 percent were still exercising an hour a day after two years, and they were the only ones who kept the weight off. Unfortunately, you don't get credit for the exercise you did in the past — you must continue with the increased activity or the weight will return.

I recommend that you view your weight problem as a strategic problem. What strategies do you need to implement to eat better and be more active? Setting goals at the beginning of the week and reviewing them at the end will allow you to experiment until you find strategies that work for you. The change in activity required is substantial, but so is the payoff.

Better together

If you only cut calories to lose weight, without increasing your physical activity, you may lose muscle as well as body fat, and your health won't benefit as much.

Activity — especially exercise — increases the number of calories you burn, not just during the activity but afterwards as well. The longer and harder the activity, the longer your energy expenditure remains elevated, burning calories.

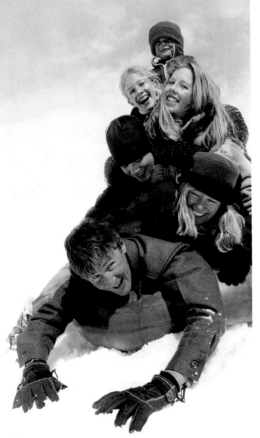

3,500 calories

Eat 3,500 fewer calories in a week and you'll lose 1 pound. But throw in some activity — a brisk walk, some vigorous gardening, a round of golf (walking), whatever you like — to burn an extra 500 calories a day, and you'll lose another pound.

Burning calories helps, and the more you burn, the more weight you lose.

Physical activity and exercise

Physical activity is any movement you do that burns calories — from gardening to walking to stretching during a work break.

Exercise is a planned, repetitive form of physical activity that improves fitness — such as swimming laps, bicycling, brisk walking and lifting weights.

All physical activity you do throughout the day, even if it's not a form of structured exercise, can help you lose weight. And the more active you are, the more calories you'll burn. For example, brisk walking for an hour might burn 300 calories. Jogging for that same hour could burn more than twice that. The more intense the activity, the more calories you burn in the same amount of time.

Now there's a balancing act here. You have to consider what's realistic for you given such constraints as your schedule and your health.

And if you're starting from a relatively low level of fitness, you'll need to ease into increased activity so you don't burn out or injure yourself. That could limit your ability to be active, which would hurt your weight-loss efforts. Not what you want to do. So it's important to strike a healthy balance.

But don't let these considerations be an excuse for not being active. If you want to lose weight, being active is a key part of the formula.

The bottom line — do whatever you can to increase your daily physical activity, and for added weight loss (and health benefits), exercise.

Do you need to see a doctor?

If you're middle-aged or older, are significantly overweight, or have been inactive for several years, talk to your doctor before increasing your activity level. Your doctor can help you choose activities that are safe and beneficial for you.

Consult your doctor before you start exercising if any of the following apply:

+ You have a heart condition and your activity should be medically supervised.
+ You have a family history of heart-related problems before age 55.
+ You have a medical condition requiring a doctor's care.
+ You smoke.
+ You get breathless or experience chest pain after mild exertion.
+ You have frequent dizzy spells.
+ You have severe joint, muscle, ligament or tendon problems.
+ You've been told to reduce your physical activity for any reason.
+ You're taking medications, such as insulin, that may require adjustment if you exercise.

Start where you are

It's been said that the best form of physical activity for losing weight is the one you'll do, and the best time to do it is whenever you can. That's a good place to start. Here are tips for building an activity program that will help you lose weight:

+ **Walk before you run.** Enthusiasm about your new activity program may lead you to the "terrible toos" — too much, too hard, too often, too soon. This all-or-nothing approach is a recipe for discouragement, not to mention injury. Start slowly and gradually build up.

+ **Do what you enjoy.** If you want an exercise program that you'll stay with, the program should be filled with activities that are fun for you. Many forms of activity can increase your fitness level. The trick is choosing ones that also stimulate and entertain you. Don't train for a marathon if you dislike running!

+ **Pick a time and stick with it.** Schedule specific times to exercise, whether it's for a two-hour workout or at short, regular intervals. Write the times (in pen, so you can't change it!) in your day calendar or journal **JOT IT** ▸, and remind yourself with Post-it notes or a watch alarm — don't try to fit exercise into your "spare time." If you don't make it a priority, exercise will be pushed aside for other concerns.

+ **Warm up.** Give yourself time to warm up before exercise with easy walking and gentle stretching. Then speed up activity to a pace you can continue without getting overly tired. As your stamina improves, gradually increase the amount of time you exercise. Aim for at least 30 to 60 minutes of exercise most days. Cool down after exercise.

+ **Break things up if you have to.** You don't have to do all your exercise or physical activity at one time. Ten minutes of exercise three times a day may be almost as beneficial as one 30-minute session.

+ **Find an exercise buddy.** Knowing that someone is waiting for you to show up in the park or at the gym is a powerful incentive. Working out with a friend, co-worker or family member can bring a new level of motivation to your workouts. Plan family outings that include hiking, swimming or skiing. Personal trainers also can be helpful, as can taking an exercise class.

+ **Talk to your family.** You'll need your family's help to make time to exercise and to provide support on the days when you're feeling sluggish. Ideally, you'll be able to do things together, increasing everyone's activity.

+ **Listen to your body.** Exercise shouldn't cause discomfort or pain. If you feel pain, shortness of breath, dizziness or nausea, take a break — you may be pushing yourself too hard. On days that you're generally not feeling well, take a day or two off and resume as soon as you can.

+ **Problem solve.** Set activity goals at the beginning of each week and review them at the end of the week. Did you achieve your goals? If so, congratulate yourself and set new goals for the following week. If not, ask yourself if the goals you set were realistic. If not, set realistic goals for the following week.

+ **Use a realistic strategy.** If you aren't a morning person, setting the alarm clock for 4:30 a.m. to get up and exercise just isn't going to work. Try right after work. If your knees can't handle jogging, try cycling or swimming.

Mild muscle soreness following exercise is common, especially if you're trying a new activity. This type of soreness should disappear in a day or two, and mild activity can help the process. Pain during exercise sends a different signal — it can be a warning sign of impending injury. Most of these injuries result from trying to do too much, too hard, too soon.

Use an activity journal

A journal is the best way to keep track of daily activities. **JOT IT** ▸ It should function much the same as a food journal to help you stay on track.

Adding activities to your day

Take advantage of every opportunity you have to get up and move around — any movement burns calories. Here are some simple ways to get more activity into your day. Also see Chapter 18 (pages 172-179), and the Action Guide to Weight-Loss Barriers (pages 180-207).

At home

+ Stretch, walk on a treadmill, or use an exercise bike while watching TV.
+ Manually wash your car.
+ Use hand tools instead of power tools.
+ Rake leaves instead of using a blower.
+ Vacuum carpets and dust the furniture.
+ Go for a short walk before breakfast. Or schedule dinner 30 minutes earlier than normal and go for a walk afterward.
+ Walk on your treadmill while reading.
+ Walk while talking on the phone.

At work

+ Take the stairs, not the elevator, at least for the first few floors — up and down.
+ Take a walk during your lunch break.
+ Get up and visit your co-workers instead of emailing them.
+ Do stretching exercises or light calisthenics at your desk.
+ Take an activity break — get up and stretch and walk around.

+ Walk around your office while talking on the phone.
+ Use a workstation that combines a treadmill with a computer, so you can walk while working.

Out and about

+ Park a little farther from your destination and walk.
+ Bike or walk to the store.
+ Join a local recreation center.

While traveling

+ Take a walk around the terminal while you're waiting for your flight (and don't use the moving walkways!).
+ Do abdominal crunches, push-ups and stretching exercises in your hotel room. Get up a little early and walk around the neighborhood or your hotel.

+ Record how long you're active while doing household chores, errands, recreational pursuits and exercise. Although all activity helps, don't enter activity lasting less than five minutes. At the end of the day, total your time to see if you've reached your 30- to 60-minute goal.

+ Carry a watch or pedometer to measure the time you're active or the number of steps you take. Aim for 2,000-3,000 steps a day more than usual to start with and try to build to at least 10,000 steps a day.

+ Indicate the intensity of your activity (light, moderate or heavy). This is a quality of exercise that you must feel rather than measure.

+ If you think it's helpful, note your energy level, how you feel, weather conditions and terrain.

Focus on aerobics

Aerobic activities are some of the best you can do for weight loss, because their intensity is low enough that you can do them for a relatively long time, increasing calories burned. They're also a great way to help your health.

One of the neat things about aerobic activities is that there are so many to pick from. You don't have to get bored doing the same old activity. Examples of aerobic activities include low- to moderately intense:

+ Walking
+ Jogging
+ Bicycling
+ Swimming
+ Exercising with fitness equipment (such as an elliptical machine or stationary bike)
+ Water aerobics
+ Rowing
+ Cross-country skiing

A simple walking program may be your best bet to adding physical activity, especially if you haven't been particularly active. Start with slow, short walks and gradually increase the frequency, duration and intensity of your walks, in that order.

For more on burning calories, see Chapter 18 (pages 172-179).

Chapter 10
A quick review . . .
and a look ahead

You've lost weight with *Lose It!* and started a sustainable, healthy approach to weight loss with *Live It!* Now let's do a little review — and take a moment to consider the long run.

There are two parts to *The Mayo Clinic Diet. Lose It!* is for two weeks. *Live It!* is for, well, forever. But you don't want to (actually can't) lose weight forever. So . . . how does this work again?

To review: *Lose It!* introduces you to some new habits in a rather dramatic way, to push you outside your comfort zone. Remember your old habits — those things that got you where you were . . . where you don't want to be?

Lose It! is very prescriptive. Not much wiggle room. Kind of like a boot camp. Desperate times call for drastic measures. It serves a purpose, but it may not be something you could do for the rest of your life.

Live It! is a bit kinder and gentler. It's a sustainable pattern of eating and activity you can use to lose weight *and* maintain that weight loss. It's a healthy lifestyle approach perhaps best defined by the meaning of the Greek root for the word *diet* — "way of life."

Together, *Lose It!* and *Live It!* give you an immediate boost and a long-term solution. Now let's review the steps.

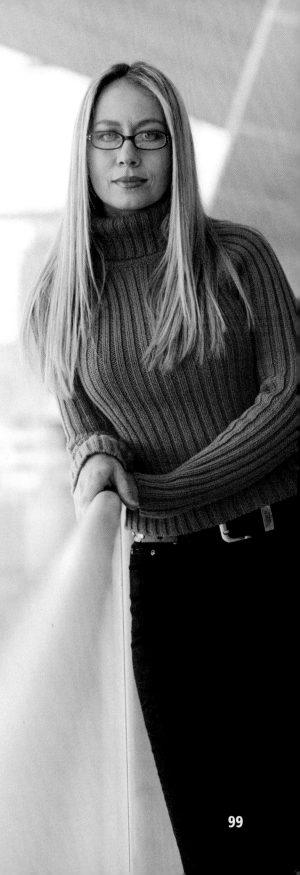

Reviewing the steps

To *Lose It!* and *Live It!*:

1 Get ready. Read Chapter 1 and make your preparations. Have on hand foods you'll want and get the necessary tools, such as a journal.
`JOT IT` ▸

2 Dive into *Lose It!* If you're ready to lose weight, you don't need to wait. Follow the 15 habits in *Lose It!* The more habits you follow, and the more closely you follow them, the more weight you're likely to lose.

3 While in *Lose It!,* prepare for *Live It!* The two phases build on each other, so you don't want a break between the two. While in *Lose It!,* read the *Live It!* chapters and:

+ Set your weight-loss goal (page 66).

+ Establish outcome or performance goals that will lead to your weight-loss goal (pages 66-67).

+ Break your goals down into intermediate steps and set deadlines.

+ Using your current weight, select your daily calorie goal (page 69).

+ Determine your daily food servings from the pyramid (pages 70-71).

+ Become familiar with serving sizes, using visual cues (pages 72-73).

+ Learn how to plan menus (pages 156-165), using your servings goals and the food lists (pages 208-235).

4 When *Lose It!* ends, use the Habit Tracker and other entries in your journal to analyze your results. `JOT IT` ▸

+ Look for what worked for you and what didn't, and why.

+ Use that information to tweak your performance goals during *Live It!*

+ Identify your strengths and weaknesses and use that information in planning for *Live It!* Play to your strengths while trying to address your weaknesses. Don't let the things you do well slip while you work on areas that need some improvement.

+ Identify what personal motivators worked best for you and use those in making your plans for *Live It!* (page 13). Keep those personal motivators in front of you.

+ Analyze your accountability. Did you have enough family or social support during *Lose It!* to be successful? What can you do to improve support? Did you weigh in regularly? Make plans to adjust what you need to during *Live It!*

+ Adapt and adjust your *Live It!* plans to suit your individual situation, your tastes and your preferences. You'll be more successful if you make your plan your own.

5 Begin *Live It!*, keeping your personal goals and motivators in front of you. This is where a notebook or journal can be invaluable. **JOT IT ▶**

6 As you *Live It!*, use the resources in Part 3 of this book for help. They'll help you plan menus (pages 156-165), build an exercise program (pages 172-179), change behaviors (pages 132-141), deal with lapses

(pages 142-155), overcome obstacles (pages 180-207), and much more.

7 At any time in *Live It!*, repeat *Lose It!* if you want an extra weight-loss bump. (But then come back to *Live It!*)

Your ultimate goal

No one wants to be on a "diet" forever. If you are, that means you're locked into a cycle of losing weight and then gaining it back. Plus, dieting is work. You've got all that planning of menus, tracking what you eat, finding ways to increase your physical activity, and monitoring your weight.

The goal of *The Mayo Clinic Diet* is to help you diet to lose weight and to find a diet (as in *way of life*) that you can enjoy for a lifetime — and without the work of "dieting." You'll have the knowledge and habits to be "close enough" in what you eat and what you do to be able to stay on track.

Over time, you may want an occasional refresher. Use these two pages for a quick review and reference guide. Now, go live *The Mayo Clinic Diet*!

Part 3 All the Extra Stuff

Lose It! and *Live It!* are the *doing* parts of *The Mayo Clinic Diet*. Part 3 gives you important support information.

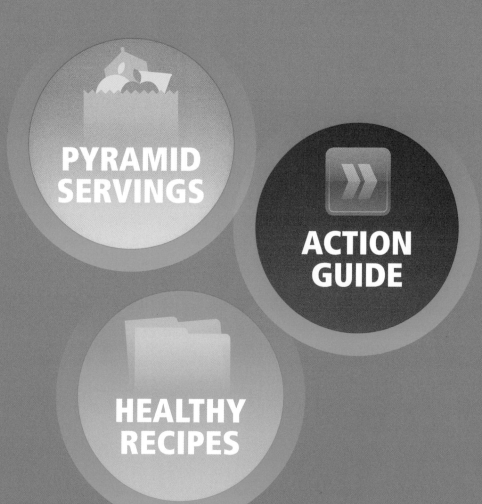

PYRAMID SERVINGS

ACTION GUIDE

HEALTHY RECIPES

Chapter 11
Finding your healthy weight

How much *should* you weigh? Well, that's not an easy question. There's no one-size-fits-all answer. The right weight for you is unique to you and dependent on a number of factors (including — but not solely — what you *want* to weigh). And, of course, your health is an important part of the equation. This chapter will help you weigh the considerations.

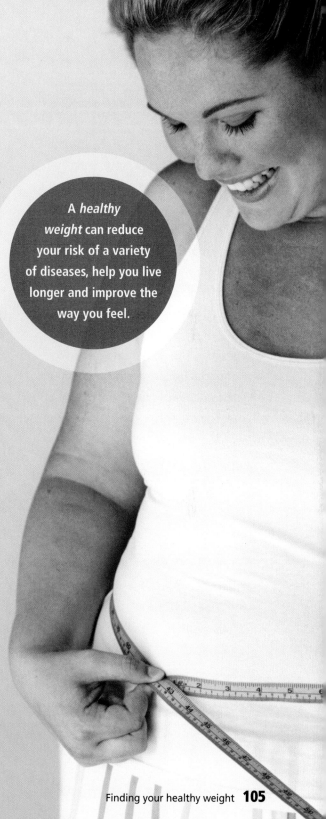

You probably already know *why* you *want* to lose weight, but *how* do you know you *need* to lose weight?

"Hey, just look at me! Isn't it obvious?" may be your answer.

Maybe. Maybe not.

Looks may play a role in determining the right weight for you. And it's a valid one — how you look helps shape your self-image, and that can affect your mental health. Looks are a valid consideration (as long as you're keeping things in realistic perspective).

But for a moment, put aside how you look in a mirror (or a swimsuit) and consider another critical factor — your health.

Being at a weight that's good for your health — what we'll call a *healthy weight* — can reduce your risk of a variety of diseases, help you live longer and improve the way you feel. And oh, it may just improve the way you feel about how you look.

A *healthy weight* can reduce your risk of a variety of diseases, help you live longer and improve the way you feel.

What is a healthy weight?

Simply put, a healthy weight means you have the right amount of body fat in relation to your overall body mass. It's a weight that allows you to feel energetic, reduces health risks, helps prevent premature aging (such as worn-out joints from carrying around too much weight) and improves your quality of life.

Stepping on the scale only tells you your total weight — including bone, muscle and fluid — not how much of your weight is fat. The scale also doesn't tell you where you're carrying that fat. In determining health risks, both of these factors are more important than is weight alone.

So how do you know if you're at a healthy weight? While there are no objective standards for what weight "looks good," there are standards for what determines a healthy weight.

The most accurate way to determine how much fat you're carrying is to have a body fat analysis. This requires a professional using a reliable method of estimation, such as weighing a person underwater or using an X-ray procedure called dual energy X-ray absorptiometry. Either method can be expensive and fairly complicated. A procedure called bioelectric impedance analysis is more widely available, but its accuracy can vary.

The most common method to determine weight-related health risk is the National Institutes of Health threefold approach:

+ Your body mass index (BMI)
+ The circumference of your waist
+ Personal medical history

Body mass index (BMI)

BMI is a tool for indicating your weight status (see the table on page 107). The mathematical calculation takes into account both your weight and height. Although BMI doesn't distinguish between fat and muscle, it more closely reflects measures of body fat than does total body weight.

Although a BMI number tends to correlate with body fat for most people,

What's your BMI?

To determine your BMI, find your height in the left column. Follow that row across to the weight nearest yours. Look at the top of that column for your approximate BMI. Or use this formula:

1 Multiply your height (in inches) by your height (in inches).
2 Divide your weight (in pounds) by the results of the first step.
3 Multiply that answer by 703. (For example, a 270-pound person, 68 inches tall, has a BMI of 41.)

	Normal		Overweight					Obese				
BMI	19	24	25	26	27	28	29	30	35	40	45	50
Height						Weight in pounds						
4'10"	91	115	119	124	129	134	138	143	167	191	215	239
4'11"	94	119	124	128	133	138	143	148	173	198	222	247
5'0"	97	123	128	133	138	143	148	153	179	204	230	255
5'1"	100	127	132	137	143	148	153	158	185	211	238	264
5'2"	104	131	136	142	147	153	158	164	191	218	246	273
5'3"	107	135	141	146	152	158	163	169	197	225	254	282
5'4"	110	140	145	151	157	163	169	174	204	232	262	291
5'5"	114	144	150	156	162	168	174	180	210	240	270	300
5'6"	118	148	155	161	167	173	179	186	216	247	278	309
5'7"	121	153	159	166	172	178	185	191	223	255	287	319
5'8"	125	158	164	171	177	184	190	197	230	262	295	328
5'9"	128	162	169	176	182	189	196	203	236	270	304	338
5'10"	132	167	174	181	188	195	202	209	243	278	313	348
5'11"	136	172	179	186	193	200	208	215	250	286	322	358
6'0"	140	177	184	191	199	206	213	221	258	294	331	368
6'1"	144	182	189	197	204	212	219	227	265	302	340	378
6'2"	148	186	194	202	210	218	225	233	272	311	350	389
6'3"	152	192	200	208	216	224	232	240	279	319	359	399
6'4"	156	197	205	213	221	230	238	246	287	328	369	410

Source: National Institutes of Health, 1998
*Asians with a BMI of 23 or higher may have an increased risk of health problems.

it's not always a good match. Some people may have a high BMI but relatively little body fat. For example, an athlete may be 6 feet 3 inches tall and weigh 230 pounds, giving him a BMI of 29 — well above the classification of healthy weight. But he's not overweight because training has turned most of his weight into lean muscle mass.

By the same token, there may be some people who have a BMI in the "healthy" range but who carry a high percentage of body fat. For most people, though, BMI provides a fairly accurate approximation of health risk as it relates to their weight.

Waist measurement

Many conditions associated with excess weight, such as high blood pressure, abnormal levels of blood fats, coronary artery disease, stroke, diabetes and certain types of cancer, are influenced by the location of body fat.

Fat distribution can be described as apple-shaped or pear-shaped. If you carry most of your fat around your waist or upper body, you're referred to as apple-shaped. If most of your fat is around your hips and thighs or lower body, you're pear-shaped.

In general, when it comes to your health, it's better to have a pear shape than an apple shape. If you have an apple shape, you carry fat in and around your abdominal organs. Fat in and around your abdomen increases your risk of developing disease. If you have a pear shape, your risks aren't as high.

To determine whether you're carrying too much weight around your middle, measure your waist. Find the highest point on each hipbone and measure around your body just above those points. A measurement exceeding 40 inches in men or 35 inches in women indicates an apple shape and increased health risks.

The table on page 109 can help you determine whether to be concerned about your waistline.

Although these cutoffs of 40 and 35 inches are useful guides, there's

Is your health at risk?

If your BMI is less than 18.5, talk with your doctor. You may be at risk of health conditions associated with a low body weight. A BMI of 18.5 to 24.9 is considered a healthy range, but Asians with a BMI of 23 or more may have an increased risk of health problems. If your BMI is higher, see below.

Weight-related risk of disease

IF Your body mass index (BMI) is ▼		& Your waist measurement is ▼	
		Women: 35 inches or less Men: 40 inches or less	Women: Over 35 inches Men: Over 40 inches
Overweight	25-29.9	Increased risk	High risk
Obese	30-34.9 35-39.9	High risk Very high risk	Very high risk Very high risk
Extreme obesity	40 or over	Extremely high risk	Extremely high risk

Source: National Institutes of Health, 2000

nothing magic about them. It's enough to know that the bigger the waistline, the greater your health risks.

Medical history

Your BMI and waist measurement numbers don't give you the full picture of your weight status. A complete evaluation of your medical history also is important. In talking with your doctor about your weight, consider:

+ **Do you have a family history of obesity, cardiovascular disease, diabetes, high blood pressure or sleep apnea?** This may mean increased risk for you.

+ **Have you gained considerable weight since high school?** Even people with normal BMIs may be at increased risk of weight-related conditions if they've gained more than 10 pounds since young adulthood.

+ **Do you have a health condition, such as high blood pressure or type 2 diabetes, that would improve if you lost weight?**

+ **Do you smoke cigarettes or engage in little physical activity?** These factors can compound the risk represented by excess weight.

BMI and waist measurement are snapshots of your current weight. The medical history helps reveal your risk of being overweight or of developing weight-related diseases.

So what's your healthy weight?

If your BMI shows that you're not overweight, if you're not carrying too much weight around your abdomen, and if you answered no to all of the medical history questions, there's probably little health advantage to changing your weight. (But you may still improve your health through a healthy diet and physical activity.)

If your BMI is between 25 and 30 or your waist measurement exceeds healthy guidelines, and you answered yes to one or more of the medical history questions, you'll probably benefit from losing a few pounds. Talk to your doctor before you start to lose weight. And if your BMI is 30 or more, you're considered obese. Losing weight should improve your health and reduce your risk of weight-related illnesses.

Now if your analysis shows that you're at a healthy weight, but you're still dissatisfied with the way you look, then you've got some thinking to do. If you're at the middle or upper end of a healthy BMI, there's probably little risk to losing a few pounds. But if you're at the lower end of a healthy BMI range, and losing weight would push you into the underweight category (less than 18.5), then losing weight may put your health at risk.

Why am I overweight?

The simple answer to why anyone is overweight is more calories consumed than burned for a long enough time to build up excess body fat. But what's the "why" behind the why? A number of factors can play a role.

+ **Lifestyle factors.** Eating high-calorie foods, eating larger portions, more sedentary jobs, and increased use of labor-saving devices can all pack on the pounds.

+ **Genetic factors.** Evidence suggests that obesity runs in some families, but the role genes play is unclear. Scientists believe that obesity is more likely the result of a complex interaction between genes and environment. This means that although you may have a genetic predisposition to being overweight, it's not fate. Ultimately, your weight is determined by how you interact with physical and social factors.

+ **Psychological factors.** People sometimes overeat to cope with problems or to deal with emotions such as boredom, sadness and frustration. In some people, a psychiatric illness called binge-eating disorder may contribute to obesity.

+ **Other factors.** These factors may contribute to weight gain but generally aren't enough in and of themselves to lead to obesity:

▸ **Age** — As you get older, the amount of muscle in your body tends to decrease, lowering metabolism. In addition, people tend to be less active as they get older. Both result in fewer calories burned.

▸ **Stopping smoking** — Many smokers gain some weight after stopping smoking, but the benefits of stopping smoking outweigh whatever health risks may result from the weight gain.

▸ **Pregnancy** — Some women may gain more weight than recommended during a pregnancy and may retain it afterward.

▸ **Medications and illnesses** — Corticosteroids, tricyclic antidepressants, anticonvulsants, insulin and hormones may cause weight gain. Sometimes, alternative medications can be used. Only rarely can obesity can be traced to an endocrine disorder, such as low thyroid function or Cushing's syndrome. Medical conditions can sometimes interfere with activity, making weight gain more likely.

Chapter 12
Understanding nutrition and weight control

Carbohydrates, fats, protein . . . oh my!
Sounds like a lot to keep track of. But more than anything,
at its core, weight is about *energy* — and the balance
between what you take in when you eat and what you burn
through physical activity. This chapter gives some depth to
that relationship.

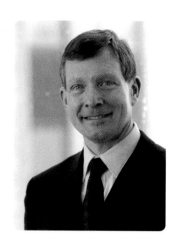

Michael Jensen, M.D.
Endocrinology

A pound of fat will provide you with 3,500 calories. You can put this in perspective by calculating about how many calories you burn a day. Your basal metabolic rate (BMR) is the number of calories a day you would burn if you lay in bed doing nothing. Because very few people are that sedentary, almost everyone burns more than this. The range of "extra" calories above BMR that we commonly see in normal adults is 20 to 75%. That means that someone with a BMR of 1,500 calories a day probably really burns somewhere between 1,800 and 2,600 calories a day.

You can get a rough estimate your own BMR by multiplying your weight by 9 to 12 calories per pound. And if you know how many minutes you walk each day, you can also calculate about how many calories you expend walking — the most common way we burn extra calories (see page 179).

Most women burn 1,700 to 2,200 calories a day and most men somewhere between 2,000 and 2,600. Now the 3,500 calories in a pound of fat can be put in perspective. It's more calories than most of us burn in an entire day — and for some women, two days! In order to lose 1 pound of fat a week, the average woman would have to reduce calorie intake by one-fourth and the average man by one-fifth. That's a lot of food to not eat just to lose a pound of fat.

It's also why reducing body fat shouldn't be looked at as a short-term goal but a long-term process.

All living things need energy to grow and develop, to function properly and, in short, to survive. Your body has a constant demand for energy. You replenish energy with the food you eat.

Weight is all about the balance between energy added through diet and energy burned through activity. This energy balance equation is a basic principle of weight control.

Food energy is measured in units called calories. It's easy to find lists of foods and the calories they contain. Energy burned in activity is also measured in calories, and there are lists to show you how many calories you can burn by doing certain activities. This knowledge is helpful in assessing your own energy balance and achieving or maintaining a healthy weight.

Tracking calories-in and calories-out in a journal is helpful in weight loss. **JOT IT** ▸ This may at first seem like a lot of work, but it's not necessarily something you have to do forever. With practice, you can get to the point where you can keep your energy flow in balance without tracking it.

Dietary sources of energy

The food you eat supplies many types of macronutrients, which provide the energy your body needs to function. These macronutrients include carbohydrates, fats and proteins. Other nutrients, such as vitamins and minerals, don't provide calories but help the body with chemical reactions. Food is also a source of water, fiber and other essential substances.

Carbohydrates

Carbohydrates can be simple or complex. Simple carbohydrates are the sugars found in fruits, honey, milk and milk products. They also include sugars added during food processing and refining. Simple carbohydrates are absorbed quickly for energy.

Complex carbohydrates, also known as starches, are found primarily in whole grains, pasta, potatoes, beans and vegetables. Digestion is required to change complex carbohydrates into simple sugars. Complex carbohydrates contain many vitamins and minerals as well as fiber.

During processing, complex carbohydrates may be refined, removing many important nutrients and their benefits.

Fats

Fats are a natural component of various foods, and they come in different forms. The oils used in cooking are a form of fat. Fats are also found in foods of animal origin, such as meat, dairy, poultry and fish, and in such common foods as avocados, nuts and olives. Fats are a major source of energy (calories) and also help your body absorb some vitamins.

Proteins

Proteins build and repair body structures, produce body chemicals, carry nutrients to your cells and help regulate body processes. Excess proteins also provide calories. Proteins are composed of basic elements called amino acids. There are two types of amino acids: those your body can generate (nonessential amino acids) and those that only can be obtained from the food you eat (essential amino acids).

What's a calorie?

Calories can be used to measure any kind of energy, but people most often associate the term with nutrition. One calorie is the amount of energy required to raise the temperature of 1 gram of water by 1 degree Celsius (1.8 F).

Because that's such a small unit of measure, food energy is measured in kilocalories (1,000 calories). The numbers you see on nutrition labels are still marked as calories, because in nutrition, calorie and kilocalorie have become synonymous.

Vitamins

Many foods contain vitamins, such as A, B complex, C, D, E and K. Vitamins help your body use carbohydrates, fats and proteins. They also help produce blood cells, hormones, genetic material and chemicals for the nervous system. Deficiencies lead to various diseases.

During processing, foods can lose nutrients. Manufacturers sometimes enrich or fortify the processed food and add back nutrients. Fresh, natural foods, though, contain vitamins in their natural, preferred state.

Minerals

Minerals such as calcium, magnesium and phosphorus are important to the health of your bones and teeth. Sodium, potassium and chloride, commonly referred to as electrolytes, help regulate the water and chemical balance in your body. Your body needs smaller amounts of minerals such as iron, iodine, zinc, copper, fluoride, selenium and manganese, commonly referred to as trace minerals.

Water

It's easy to take water for granted, but it's a vital nutritional requirement. Many foods, especially fruits, contain a lot of water. Water plays a role in nearly every major body function. It regulates body temperature, carries nutrients and oxygen to cells via the bloodstream and helps carry away waste. Water also helps cushion joints and protects organs and tissues.

Fiber

Fiber is the part of plant foods that your body doesn't absorb. The two main types of fiber are soluble and insoluble, and fiber-rich foods usually contain both.

Foods high in soluble fiber include citrus fruits, apples, pears, plums and prunes, legumes (dried beans and peas), oatmeal and oat bran, and barley. Soluble fiber helps lower blood cholesterol, slows the rise in blood sugar and adds bulk to stools.

Insoluble fiber is found in many vegetables, wheat bran, and whole-grain breads, pasta and cereals. Insoluble fiber also adds bulk to stool, stimulates the gastrointestinal tract, and helps prevent constipation.

Where the calories come from

Carbohydrates, fats and proteins are the types of nutrients that contain calories, and that means they're the main energy sources for your body. The amount of energy each nutrient provides varies.

+ Carbohydrates are the food nutrients that your body uses first. During digestion, they're released into your bloodstream and converted into glucose, or blood sugar. When there's a demand, the glucose is absorbed immediately into your body's cells to provide energy.

If there's no immediate demand, glucose can be stored in your liver and muscles. When these storage sites become full, excess glucose is converted into fatty acids and stored in fat tissue for later use.

+ Fats are an extremely concentrated form of energy and pack the most calories. When digested, they're broken down into fatty acids, which are also used for energy or for other body processes.

If there's an excess of fatty acids, a small quantity can be stored in your muscles, but most of them are stored in fat tissue. There's virtually no limit to how much fat your body can store.

+ Proteins have many responsibilities but can also supply energy for physical activity. This can happen if you consume too few calories, eat

Food sources of energy

Fats supply more calories per gram than do carbohydrates and proteins combined. Many people are surprised that alcohol can be such a high source of calories.

Nutrient	Calories (per gram)
Fats	9
Alcohol	7
Carbohydrates	4
Proteins	4

excess protein, or if you're involved in prolonged physical activity. Any excess calories from protein are converted into fat and stored.

Vitamins, minerals, water and fiber don't contain calories. However, they're still vital to your health and well-being. When they're lacking from your diet, you increase your risk of serious illness. Other substances in food, such as cholesterol, don't provide calories either.

Your energy account

The energy needs of your body can be looked at like a bank account. Lots of transactions take place. You have daily deposits and daily withdrawals.

Your deposits are food, with three nutrients providing the bulk of your energy: carbohydrates, fats and proteins. When you eat, you're adding calories to your energy account.

Withdrawals can be made in three ways, each of which burns calories:

+ **BMR.** Even when you're in a state of complete rest, your body is using energy to meet its basic needs, such as breathing, blood circulation, and cellular growth and repair. This energy use at rest is called your basal metabolic rate (BMR). Your BMR is responsible for the greatest demand on your energy account — generally, one-half to two-thirds of your total energy expenditure.

+ **Thermic effect of food.** The energy your body uses to digest, absorb, transport and store the food you eat is known as the thermic effect of food. It takes about 10 percent of your total energy use.

+ **Physical activity.** Daily tasks such as getting dressed, brushing your teeth and other routine activities also require energy. At least 20 percent of your calorie needs go toward these activities.

The energy needs of your BMR and for digestion remain relatively steady and aren't easy to change. The best way to increase your energy withdrawal — in other words, to burn more calories — is to increase the amount of physical activity you do.

Influences on your energy account

If everyone were physically and functionally identical, it would be easy to determine the standard energy needs for all kinds of activity. But other factors affect your energy account.

Some of the factors that influence your BMR and your overall energy needs are age, body size and composition, and sex.

+ **Age.** Children and adolescents, who are in the process of developing their bones, muscles and tissues, need more calories per pound than do adults. In fact, infants need the most calories per pound of any age group because of their rapid growth and development.

As hormone levels and body composition change with age, so does your BMR. By the time you reach early middle age, your BMR and energy needs are declining, generally at a rate of 2 percent a decade.

+ **Body size and composition.** A bigger body mass requires more energy, and thus more calories, than does a smaller body mass. In addition, muscle burns more calories than does fat, so the more muscle you have in relation to fat, the higher your BMR.

Based on this principle, you can slightly increase your BMR and the amount of energy you burn by building up your muscle mass through regular physical activity.

Empty calories

Empty calories is a term applied to sugar and alcohol. They contribute calories but few other essential nutrients.

Small amounts of alcohol (up to two drinks for men, one drink for women and anyone age 65 or older) have been linked with lower risk of heart disease.

But excessive drinking can add unwanted pounds, raise blood pressure, damage your liver and increase the risk of some cancers.

One drink equals:

+ One 12-ounce regular beer (150 calories).

+ One 5-ounce glass of wine (about 100 calories).

+ One 1½-ounce shot of hard liquor (about 100 calories — mixes can add more).

- **Sex.** Men usually have less body fat and more muscle than do women of the same age and weight. This is why men generally have a higher BMR and higher energy requirements than women do.

Balancing your account

Your body weight is a physical reflection of your energy account. Daily fluctuations in weight indicate the daily changes in your account.

If you withdraw from the account approximately the same amount of energy as you deposit, your weight stays the same. If you spend more from the account than you deposit, you lose weight.

There's a magic number in this energy equation. Because 3,500 calories equals about 1 pound of body fat, you'd need to consume 3,500 excess calories to gain a pound, and you'd need to burn 3,500 calories more than you take in to lose a pound.

The tricky part is that energy needs vary from day to day. What you eat also varies. So the balance between calories consumed and calories expended is constantly shifting.

Tracking these shifts requires a bit of old-fashioned accounting — tallying up all the sources of energy income (what you eat and drink) and all the forms of energy expenditure (activity). Tracking is helpful in losing weight (and why it's part of *Lose It!*), but who has the time and energy to do it long term?

Over the long haul, it's better to think about weight control in terms of general principles — losing weight requires an energy deficit, and you create this deficit by eating fewer calories, burning more calories through physical activity, or preferably both.

The best way to do this is through practice (as in *Lose It!*) — eating healthfully and being active. Eventually, that leads to habits that will allow you to do that without even thinking about it that much — in other words, adopting a healthy lifestyle (as in *Live It!*).

Reducing calories tends to figure more prominently than does physical activity during the initial stages of weight loss. But as you work toward a healthy weight, physical activity is more and more essential to reaching your goal.

Healthy weight control

Do you have to eat carrots and celery sticks and avoid even the sight of chocolate for the rest of your life in order to maintain a healthy weight?

No. In terms of energy balance, it's possible to eat any food you like and lose weight as long as the total calories you consume are less than the total calories you burn. But clearly, what you eat affects your health.

If the bulk of your diet consists of foods that are high in saturated fat, you increase your risk of cardiovascular disease and other diseases. And diets high in refined carbohydrates and low in fiber are linked to conditions such as diabetes and cardiovascular disease. In addition, if you're lacking vegetables and fruits in your diet, you're missing the health benefits of vitamins and minerals, phytochemicals and antioxidants.

The science behind it

The everyday decisions you make regarding the food you eat and the activity you do and, ultimately, the weight you carry, relate to what's called the first law of thermodynamics. This law states that energy must remain constant — it's neither created nor destroyed, but merely transferred or converted to different forms.

The calories you eat can either be converted to physical energy or stored within your body, but they can't magically disappear. All unused calories in your body become fat, regardless of where they come from. Unless you use these stored calories, either by reducing calorie intake so that your body must draw on reserves for energy or by increasing physical activity and the amount of energy you expend, this fat will remain in your body.

In theory, the energy balance equation is simple. In practice, applying it can be a bit more complex. But as you grasp the concept of energy balance, weight control may become easier to understand. And a key point is that a healthy weight can be achieved in a way that allows you to enjoy food as well as long-term health.

Chapter 13
The Mayo Clinic Healthy Weight Pyramid

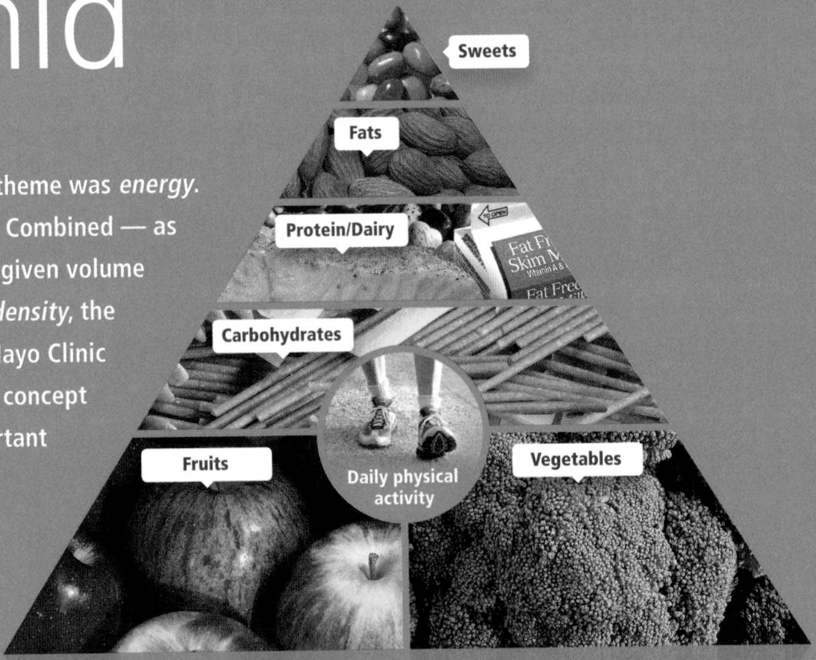

In the last chapter, the main theme was *energy*. In this chapter, think *volume*. Combined — as in the amount of energy in a given volume of food — you have *energy density*, the underlying principle of the Mayo Clinic Healthy Weight Pyramid. The concept of energy density is an important weight-loss tool.

Sweets

Fats

Protein/Dairy

Carbohydrates

Fruits

Daily physical activity

Vegetables

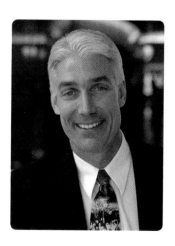

Donald Hensrud, M.D.
Preventive Medicine
and Endocrinology

If you think about what determines how much you eat, it isn't calories. You don't say to yourself, "I've eaten 500 calories, now I'm full." You eat until you're satisfied from consuming enough volume or weight of food. Therefore, if you can eat foods that provide a lot of weight and volume (bulk) but not many calories, you can feel full while losing or maintaining weight.

The Mayo Clinic Healthy Weight Pyramid is designed to do just that. Beyond weight, health is obviously important, which is why the Mayo Clinic Healthy Weight Pyramid emphasizes health-promoting choices within each of its six food groups.

Vegetables and fruits are the foundation of the Mayo Clinic Healthy Weight Pyramid. Virtually unlimited amounts of fresh or frozen veggies and fruits (not dried fruits or juices) are recommended for their beneficial effects on both weight and health. Similarly, whole-grain carbohydrates are healthier than are their refined (think white flour) counterparts, and in moderate amounts can help control weight. Lean sources of protein and dairy and heart-healthy unsaturated fats contribute to good health and good taste. Even an occasional treat is OK.

Eating to the pyramid can be effective for weight management and good health. Eating well doesn't have to be drudgery. Incorporating recommended foods and amounts in great-tasting dishes can truly be an enjoyable way to live. Bon appétit!

All foods contain a certain number of calories (energy) in a given amount (volume), and the number varies from one type of food to another.

Some foods are high in calories, even for a small amount. They're considered high in energy density. These foods include most high-fat foods, simple sugars, alcohol, fast foods, sodas, candies and processed foods. Other foods don't have many calories, even for a relatively large amount. These foods, such as vegetables and fruits, are low in energy density.

Let's look at a couple of examples. A regular candy bar might have 270 calories. A lot of calories in a small package makes for high energy density. In contrast, 1 cup of most raw vegetables contains only about 25 calories. Not many calories in a fairly large volume makes for low energy density. You could eat 11 cups of raw vegetables to get as many calories as you would from that one candy bar.

Where this helps in weight loss is that foods low in energy density typically leave you feeling satisfied on fewer calories, while foods high in energy density are less likely to fill you up — or if you do fill up on them, you've chowed down a lot of calories.

Feeling full on fewer calories may seem like a weight-loss gimmick, but the concept is backed by science. Research suggests that feeling full is strongly determined by the volume and weight of food in your stomach, not necessarily by the number of calories you eat.

Participants in several studies who switched to a diet of low-energy-density foods were able to lose significant amounts of weight. More importantly, they were able to stick to the low-energy-density diet and keep a good deal of the weight off over time, decreasing their risk of weight-related diseases.

By choosing foods with a low energy density, you can consume fewer calories while still feeling full — and lose weight. That's the heart of the Mayo Clinic Healthy Weight Pyramid.

Now let's look in more detail at the pyramid's individual sections.

Vegetables and Fruits

Vegetables and fruits share many attributes. In fact, some foods that we term vegetable are technically fruits. Both offer a wide array of flavors, textures and colors. They provide not only sensory pleasure but also many disease-fighting nutrients.

Most vegetables and fruits are low in energy density because they're high in water and fiber, which provide no calories. You can improve your diet — and actually eat more food — by eating more vegetables and fruits in place of higher calorie foods.

Vegetables

Vegetables include roots and tubers such as carrots, radishes and beets, members of the cabbage family, and salad greens such as lettuce and spinach. Other plant foods, such as tomatoes, peppers and cucumbers, are included in this group, although technically they're fruits.

One pyramid serving of vegetables contains about 25 calories. Vegetables

Less dense, more filling

Three factors play important roles in what makes vegetables and fruits less energy dense and more filling:

88% water
52 calories

+ **Water** — Most fruits and vegetables contain a lot of water, which provides volume and weight but not calories. A small grapefruit, for example, is about 90 percent water and has just 64 calories. Carrots are about 88 percent water and have only 52 calories in 1 cup (more than two pyramid servings!).
+ **Fat** — Most fruits and vegetables do not contain a lot of fat. Fat raises energy density. One teaspoon of butter contains almost the same number of calories as 2 cups of broccoli!
+ **Fiber** — Fiber is the part of plant-based foods that your body doesn't absorb. The high-fiber content in foods such as vegetables, fruits and whole grains provides bulk to your diet, so it makes you feel full sooner. The fiber also takes longer to digest, making you feel full longer.

contain no cholesterol, are low in fat and sodium and high in dietary fiber. They're also high in essential minerals such as potassium and magnesium, and contain beneficial plant chemicals known as phytochemicals.

Fresh vegetables are best, but frozen vegetables are good, too. Most canned vegetables are high in sodium because sodium is used as a preservative in the canning process. If you use canned vegetables, look for labels that indicate that no salt has been added, or rinse them before use.

Fruits

Most food that contains seeds surrounded by an edible layer is generally considered a fruit. In North America, fruits such as apples, oranges, peaches and plums, and slightly more exotic fruits such as mangos and papayas, are commonly available. These foods taste sweet or sweet-tart and are often eaten for snacks or desserts.

Like vegetables, fruits are great sources of fiber, vitamins, minerals and other phytochemicals. One

pyramid serving equals about 60 calories and is virtually fat-free, so fruits can help you control your weight and reduce your risk of weight-related diseases.

Fresh fruit is best, but frozen fruits with no added sugar and fruits canned in their own juice or water also are excellent. Because of processing, fruit juice and dried fruits, such as raisins and prunes, can be a concentrated source of calories — they have a higher energy density. Use them sparingly.

Carbohydrates

Carbohydrates include a wide range of foods that are major energy sources for your body. One pyramid serving is about 70 calories. Most carbohydrates are plant-based. They include grain products, such as breads, cereals and pasta, and certain starchy vegetables, such as potatoes and corn. Which kind should you focus on?

Think of all the carbohydrate-containing foods laid out in a line. At one end are whole wheat, oats and brown rice. In the middle, white flour, white rice,

WHAT IF YOU HAVE HEALTH CONCERNS?

You feel like a snack and there's an orange handy. But you've avoided fruit because you've got diabetes, and you're concerned about what that orange will do to your blood sugar.

What should you do?

That depends on you. If you're overweight, closely following the calorie and activity guidelines of this book will have you losing excess pounds. And if you're losing weight, eating fruit won't necessarily affect your blood sugar in a negative way.

Likely, you'll be just fine following the eating principles of the Mayo Clinic Healthy Weight Pyramid, which allows unlimited fruits and vegetables. But, you still need to monitor your blood sugar to see how eating by the principles of the pyramid affects you.

The Mayo Clinic Healthy Weight Pyramid is suitable for the vast majority of people, including most people with health concerns such as diabetes and high triglycerides. But, as with any valid eating program, it's not a one-size-fits-all approach. You may need to adapt it to your specific health situation or needs. For example, if you don't tolerate certain foods, don't eat them.

The Mayo Clinic Healthy Weight Pyramid has enough flexibility to allow modifications, so work with your doctor or a registered dietitian to find out how to apply the principles of the pyramid in a way that works best for you.

potatoes and pastas. And at the other end are highly processed products — cookies, candies and soft drinks.

The foods in that spectrum incorporate all three kinds of carbohydrates: fiber, starch and sugar. It's not hard to point to the healthy and less healthy ends — less refined whole grains on one end, highly refined sugar on the other.

The health pros and cons of many items in the middle aren't so clear. Rice, pasta, bread and potatoes can all shift depending on how they're processed and served.

Consider, for example, white and whole-wheat (whole-grain) breads. Both begin as nutrient-rich whole grains, as do both white and brown rice. During

What about low-carb diets?

Many diets promote low-carbohydrate foods for weight loss. These diets claim that carbohydrates stimulate insulin secretion, which promotes body fat. So, the logic goes, reducing carbohydrates will reduce body fat.

As a matter of fact, carbohydrates do stimulate insulin secretion immediately after they're consumed, but this is a normal process that allows carbohydrates to be absorbed into cells.

People who gain weight on high-carbohydrate diets do so because they're eating excess calories. Excess calories from any source will cause weight gain. Furthermore, some low-carbohydrate diets restrict grains, fruits and vegetables and emphasize protein and dairy products, which can be high-calorie and loaded with saturated fat and cholesterol.

Recent studies confirm that the most important factor in weight change is total calories, not where they come from.

processing, however, the grain's bran and germ are refined away, taking with them many of their vitamins and almost all of their fiber. That's why it's wise to choose whole-grain breads, pastas and cereals, and to serve brown rice instead of white.

Similarly, the edible skins so often removed from potatoes and sweet potatoes are full of nutrients and fiber.

When picking carbohydrates, the key word is *whole*. Generally, the less refined a carbohydrate food, the better it is for you.

Protein and Dairy

Protein is essential to human life. Your skin, bone, muscle and organ tissues are made up of protein, and it's present in your blood, too. Protein is often associated with foods of animal origin, but it's also found in plants.

Foods rich in protein and relatively low in fat and saturated fat include legumes, fish, skinless poultry and lean meat. Whole-milk dairy products are good sources of protein and calcium but are high in saturated fat. Low-fat or skim milk, yogurt and cheese have the same nutritional value as the whole-milk varieties but without the fat and calories. They're relatively low in energy density, too, because they contain a lot of water.

Many cuts of chicken, turkey, beef, lamb and pork can be too high in saturated fat and cholesterol to include regularly in a healthy diet. Focus on lean cuts of meat, and remember that other everyday ingredients, including low-fat dairy products, seafood and many plant foods, furnish protein, too.

Legumes, namely beans, lentils, and peas, are an excellent source of protein because they have no cholesterol and very little fat. They're great for filling out or replacing dishes made with poultry or meat. Unlike meat, beans help lower the "bad" form of cholesterol (LDL), and the minerals they contain help control blood pressure.

Although the protein in beans is "incomplete," meaning it lacks essential amino acids that meats provide, the missing nutrients are plentiful in other plant foods, so people who lighten up on meat can easily get all they need. Among legumes, only soybeans have protein containing all the essential amino acids.

Fish and shellfish are not only fine protein sources, but some also supply omega-3 fatty acids. These can help lower triglycerides, fat particles in the blood that appear to raise the risk of heart disease. They may also help prevent dangerous heartbeat disturbances known as arrhythmias, improve immune function and help regulate blood pressure. Research suggests that most people would benefit by eating at least two servings of fish a week.

One serving from the protein and dairy group of the pyramid is 110 calories.

Fats

You may find it hard to believe, but fats are essential to the life and function of your body's cells. Really.

Along with providing reserves of stored energy, fats play a role in the immune system, help maintain cell structure and play a role in the regulation of many other body processes. Deposits of fat tissue protect and insulate vital body organs. In short, you need some fat in your diet.

But not all fats are created equal (see "Fats: The good and the bad," page 29), and that's where the pyramid can help guide your choices.

Studies over the past two decades have confirmed that people who replace much of the animal fat in their meals with liquid vegetable oils stand a good chance of bringing down their blood cholesterol levels, lowering their risk of cardiovascular disease.

Other findings suggest that people who favor foods made with liquid oils, such as canola and olive oils, over ones with solid shortenings and margarines may derive similar health benefits.

A key point — the pyramid's fat group recommendations address only the fats that are typically *added* to a day's meals, not the fat within other foods (such as meats). These added fats

include salad dressings, cooking oils, butter, and high-fat plant foods, such as avocados, olives, seeds and nuts.

Most of these high-fat plant foods are good for you. Nuts, for instance, contain a type of fat — monounsaturated fat — that helps keep hearts and arteries free of harmful deposits. They're also a good source of protein, and depending on the type, they also deliver many other key nutrients, including thiamin, niacin, folate, selenium, zinc and vitamin E.

All nuts are also a source of flavonoids, a group of antioxidants that protect blood vessels and other cells from damage, reducing the risk of heart disease and certain cancers.

But while nuts and vegetable oils may be beneficial, they're still high in calories. A tablespoon of peanut butter weighs in at nearly 100 calories and a tablespoon of olive oil at 140. Fats contain approximately 45 calories in a pyramid serving and are a high-energy-density food. For that reason, all fats, including the healthier ones, should be consumed sparingly.

Where does alcohol fit?

Alcohol is a fairly concentrated source of calories — about 7 calories per gram (topped only by fat) — but has no nutritional value. For that reason, it's included under sweets in the Mayo Clinic Healthy Weight Pyramid.

Consider it a treat. You don't have to eliminate it under the *Live It!* phase of *The Mayo Clinic Diet*, but limit your consumption to an average of 75 calories a day over the course of a week.

→ For more on alcohol, see page 119.

And what about the fats contained within other foods, such as meats, seafoods and many dairy products? These are limited through the serving recommendations under the other pyramid food groups.

Sweets

Foods in the sweets group include sugar-sweetened beverages, such as regular sodas and fruit drinks, candies, cakes, cookies, pies, doughnuts and other desserts. And don't forget the table sugar you add to cereal, fruit and beverages.

Foods in the sweets group are a high source of calories, mostly from sugar and fat, and are high in energy density, yet they offer little in terms of nutrition. You don't have to give up these foods entirely. But be smart about your selections and portion sizes.

The pyramid recommends limiting sweets to 75 calories a day. For practicality, average that over a week. Where possible, select better dessert choices, such as a small amount of dark chocolate or low-fat frozen yogurt.

Physical activity

The Mayo Clinic Healthy Weight Pyramid is not just about food. At the center of the pyramid is a circle that recognizes the important role physical activity plays in weight loss and health.

The pyramid recommends 30 to 60 minutes of moderately vigorous physical activity on most days of the week. For more on how to accomplish that, see Chapter 9 (pages 90-97) and Chapter 18 (pages 172-179).

Chapter 14
How to change behaviors

Newborn babies are remarkably direct about food. When they're hungry, they cry. When they're full, they refuse to eat. You probably don't act that way now. Chances are, over time you've learned eating habits in response to factors other than hunger, factors often triggered by a preoccupied brain rather than an empty stomach. But you can change those habits and learn new behaviors.

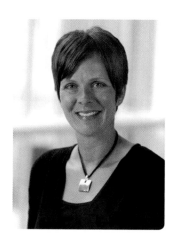

Paula Ricke
Health and Wellness
Specialist

Congratulations on being here at this moment, reading this book, and taking another step toward a lifelong commitment to healthy living. You are traveling down your wellness journey: a journey of successes and challenges as well as self-discovery.

Anticipate obstacles on your wellness journey. Life happens. Even the most thought-out behavior change plans will usually require some adjustments along the way. One off day does not mean failure. It simply means you get back on track and face tomorrow with renewed confidence in your ability to be successful.

Be realistic with your behavior change. It took months or even years to form your current behaviors, so why should you think you can change those behaviors overnight? You are striving to make permanent lifestyle changes. That is no easy task. It will take an adequate amount of time for your new habits to feel natural. Keep a positive attitude and make small, doable lifestyle changes.

Reward yourself. Be supportive and encouraging of yourself along your wellness journey. Focus on and reward successes, no matter how small you feel they are. Every success is a victory.

This chapter will give you many tips on how to prepare for and be successful with behavior change. Make the commitment today to leading a healthy lifestyle. The journey is *yours* to succeed at, so enjoy!

The only proven formula for achieving and maintaining a healthy weight — eat less and move more — sounds simple. But anyone who's tried to lose weight knows that it's more challenging than it sounds.

What gets in the way? Often, it's learned behaviors — some unintentional.

Physical symptoms, emotions, social pressure, conditioned thinking, lack of awareness, and other factors influence behaviors. To lose weight, you need to target those underlying factors, not just what you eat or do.

Preparing for change

Because everyone is different, changing a behavior is a highly individualized process. The method, timing and pace of change vary from one person to the next. As you contemplate making a change in your life, here are some general principles to guide you:

+ **It's not a race.** Sometimes, a little shock therapy can help. That's what's behind *Lose It!* It's designed to bump you off your normal course and show you that change can bring results.

But long-term change, involving basic lifestyle shifts, typically doesn't happen overnight. It takes time and dedication to unlearn unhealthy behaviors and develop new, healthy ones that lead to permanent weight loss. Plan for long-term weight loss, but feel free to repeat *Lose It!* if you need a boost and a reminder that change works.

+ **Don't overreact to the scale.** Weighing yourself regularly can help in weight loss, but don't let daily variations in your weight upset you. They may be just fluid changes. You have better control over what you eat and what you do than over numbers on the scale, so concentrate on those actions as your goal.

+ **Anticipate a lapse.** There will be days when you eat more or move less than you intended. That's what's called a lapse, and it's inevitable that you'll occasionally lapse.

But it's important not to use a lapse as an excuse to give up. Have a plan for such occasions. See Chapter 15 (pages 142-155) for more on lapses.

Strengthen your resolve

Many people stay on a diet for only a week or two before giving up. Often, they've been unable to change unhealthy behaviors that weaken their commitment. They may have been unable to resist favorite high-calorie foods. They may have overdone their exercise program.

To achieve and maintain a healthy weight, you need to identify unhealthy behaviors and work to change them permanently. That takes commitment. That takes motivation. To strengthen your resolve to change before you start taking action, see chapters 1 and 15 and review the motivators in *Lose It!*

How to change behavior

Behavior change doesn't happen by accident. If you want to make lasting changes to your eating and activity habits, you need a plan.

There are many strategies for how to change to healthier behaviors. Everyone has his or her own approach and his or her own pace for making changes. And it's likely that you won't follow the same plan for every change you want to make. What's important is that you clearly identify and examine the behaviors that interfere with your ability to lose weight and find healthy ways to deal with them.

Here's a list of steps that you may take to change an unhealthy behavior:

1. **List those behaviors that you feel are unhealthy.** Common examples include eating too quickly, snacking throughout the day instead of eating regular meals, eating when you're under stress, and skipping your walk when the weather's not perfect or if the television beckons.

2. **Select one behavior that you would like to change.** Trying to change all the behaviors on your list at once can feel overwhelming and increase the chance that you won't be successful. Focus on changing one behavior at a time.

Put the brakes on stress

Stress can take a toll on your health, cause weight gain and create sleep troubles — all of which can lead to even more stress and derail your weight-loss plans. To stay on track through stressful times, try this four-step strategy:

1. **Take stock of your stressors.** When you're feeling overwhelmed or upset, jot down the particular circumstances in a journal **JOT IT ▶** or notebook. Realize that stress can be caused by external factors — environment, family relations or unpredictable events — as well as by internal factors — negative attitudes, unrealistic expectations or perfectionism.

2. **Examine your stressors.** Try to identify the problem at its root. Then ask yourself, "Can I change this situation?" or "Can I improve my ability to cope with this situation?" For example, if you always find yourself stressed when deciding what to wear to certain social events, ask yourself why that is. Is it because you don't like your clothes or because you're worried about how someone or some group will judge you? Once you know what's at the root of your stress, you can take steps to deal with it.

3. **Evaluate your responsibilities.** Are you overcommitted, either at home, at work, or at both? If so, can you delegate some of your tasks? Can others assist you? Can you say no to new responsibilities? Assess and monitor your daily and weekly responsibilities and do your best not to overextend yourself.

4. **Learn to relax.** Develop a strategy that helps you relax when you find yourself becoming stressed (better yet, be proactive and practice it daily to prevent stress). Proven stress-reduction strategies include exercise, deep breathing and muscle relaxation techniques, as well as a good laugh. Any or all of these options generally provide a positive outlet for stress so that you can stay on track with your weight-loss program.

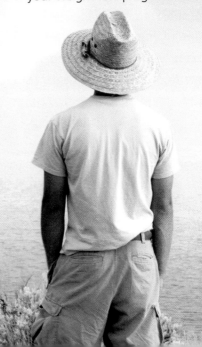

3. **As you think of strategies for change, consider how you developed the behavior.** Are there underlying causes for the behavior that also need to be addressed? For example, is your all-day snacking related to constant stress? What benefit do you get from the behavior? Are there healthier ways to obtain this benefit? What are the negative consequences of this behavior? Identifying these factors can help outline the reasons for change.

4. **Brainstorm ways to change this behavior.** Think of five to seven possible solutions, then decide on one strategy that you feel is practical and doable.

   Locking yourself out of the kitchen and carrying no money with you are two ways to prevent snacking, but they aren't realistic. Taking time over your noon hour to eat a healthy lunch and exercise is more realistic. Retain your other strategies as backups.

5. **Devise a plan to promote this strategy.** How will you go about

making sure that you have the time to eat and exercise during the day? One option might be to reserve 30 minutes to an hour every day over the lunch hour for yourself — a time when nothing else is scheduled.

6. **Identify obstacles.** Look for potential conflicts that might interfere with your strategy and make contingency plans. For example, if you can't find time to exercise, try exercising in the morning before work.

7. **Set a date for when you want to achieve your goal — making the changed behavior routine.** Establish a comfortable pace for change. Depending on what kind of behavior you're trying to change, it may take you only a few days, or it may take you several weeks or months. Jot the date down in your journal. JOT IT ▶

8. **When you reach the goal date, evaluate your success.** What worked and what didn't? What would you do differently? If you didn't reach your goal, why not? What got in your way?

9. **Consider what you need to do to maintain this change.** Reaching your goal doesn't mean that now you can stop doing what you've been working so hard at. If you start letting work responsibilities erode your lunch hour, you'll be back to your old habit of skipping lunch and snacking all day. Think about what you need to do to make your healthy behavior permanent.

10. **When ready, select another unhealthy behavior and restart the process.** Use the insight you've gained from previous behavior-change efforts to help you be successful in future attempts.

More tips for behavior change

In addition to the strategies listed above, these tips might help:

+ **Keep a food diary.** It helps to understand what causes a behavior before you try to change it. One of the best ways to do that is to keep a diary that records not just what you eat, but what triggers your eating, even when you're not hungry. Use *The Mayo Clinic Diet Journal* `JOT IT` ▸ or a notebook to track what you eat and what prompts you to eat.

+ **Enjoy your food.** When you eat, keep your mind focused on the pleasure of what you're doing. Be aware of every bite. To stay focused, you can't be doing anything else — don't read, don't watch television, just savor your food. Eating should give you pleasure, not just provide fuel for your body.

+ **Stick to your schedule.** If your diary indicates that you eat many times during the day, having a meal schedule can give you a better sense of control. This doesn't necessarily mean the traditional three meals of breakfast, lunch and dinner.

Create a schedule that's convenient and enables you to eat when you're hungry. Build flexibility into the schedule by defining half-hour or hour time frames for eating rather than setting exact times.

You may find that eating three meals and two snacks works best for you. Or perhaps six mini-meals suit your schedule better. The important thing is to stick with a routine. But don't go more than four or five hours without eating because you could become extremely hungry, causing you to overeat.

+ **Have a plan.** Try to plan what you're going to eat for the day at least one day in advance. Your decisions will depend, in part, on your daily servings goals. Planning ahead means you'll have the ingredients on hand at mealtimes and can start preparing food without delays. This helps keep you from grabbing a slice of leftover pizza when you arrive home hungry.

Planning ahead also means packing your lunch, snacks or even breakfast to take to work. This saves you from relying on vending machines or fast-food fare and from making impulsive food choices. A good rule of preparedness is always to have something ready that's healthy to munch on, such as low-calorie popcorn, cut-up vegetables or fruit.

Make it realistic and enjoyable

One of the most important steps to successful weight control is to have realistic goals and expectations. If you set your expectations too high or hold yourself to impossible goals, you're setting yourself up for failure.

Start small and take one day at a time. If you understand what's possible in the context of your everyday life and work within those parameters, you're more likely to succeed.

It's also important that you enjoy and find satisfaction in the changes you're making to your lifestyle. Consciously include satisfaction in your goal setting. A study of individuals who successfully managed their weight after completing a medically supervised weight-loss program showed that satisfaction with the amount and quality of daily activities was an important factor in success. If you don't like what you're doing to lose weight, you won't stick with the program.

As you think about your goals and expectations, look at your results from *Lose It!* Flip through your journal to find what worked and what didn't, and what you enjoyed and what you didn't. Build on that in your long-term goals.

+ **Find your eating place.** Designate an appropriate place in the house for eating, preferably at a dining table. Set the table, even if you're eating alone. Make the environment as pleasant as possible, and one without distractions. By eating in one place, you begin to associate that place, and that place only, with eating.

+ **Manage food problems.** You might trick yourself into believing that the bag of chocolate-covered peanuts you tossed into your shopping cart is for a special occasion, but once it's in the house, can you resist sampling them? Do yourself a favor. Don't buy high-calorie foods that tempt you to snack.

+ **Out of sight, out of mind.** If you do need to keep tempting foods in the house, store them where you can't see them, especially if your diary reveals that your urge to eat is triggered by visual cues.

+ **Eat from hunger, not emotion.** Food is comforting, so many people reach for food when they try to resolve a problem. People do forget what real hunger feels like. Don't eat for a few hours and see how you feel. If what you experience isn't physical hunger, don't try to comfort yourself with food. If you're tired, then rest or meditate. If you're thirsty, drink a glass of water. If you're anxious, take a walk. Stop making eating your all-purpose response to every situation.

When you have an urge to eat but you're not sure whether you're hungry, wait 15 to 30 minutes and see how you feel. Here's a clue: If you can't decide what you want to eat, chances are you're not very hungry.

+ **Stop when you're full.** No matter what you heard from your parents as a child, you don't have to finish all the food on your plate. Even if you served yourself what you considered a reasonable portion, how do you know before you start eating how much food will satisfy your hunger? Eat slowly, savor every bite and stop when you're full. If you're not good at sensing when you're full, start with a small portion on your plate.

+ **Address stress.** Eating is often associated with stress. But eating to ease stress almost always results in overeating. Finding other ways to cope with stress may prevent a lapse and unnecessary weight gain. Try these ideas (also see page 136):

  ‣ Prioritize, plan and pace your activities.
  ‣ Spend time with people who have a positive outlook and sense of humor.
  ‣ Get enough sleep to help clear your mind and make you ready for the day.
  ‣ Organize work spaces so that you know where things are.
  ‣ Get plenty of exercise.
  ‣ Take stretch breaks throughout the day.
  ‣ Do something good just for yourself or for somebody else.
  ‣ Don't feel guilty if you're not productive every minute of every day.
  ‣ Learn to delegate responsibility.
  ‣ Take a day off with no set plans.

One step at a time

We tend to be comfortable with our behaviors and habits, even if they're not always enjoyable or beneficial. They're familiar. They give order and stability to our lives.

Although change can be difficult, it's not impossible. Most people underestimate their ability to change. And changing behaviors in many small ways can add up to a big difference in lifestyle.

Here's a common dietary example: Many people have switched from drinking whole milk to skim milk. Maybe they tapered off gradually and changed to 2% milk first, or maybe they switched from one to the other in one bold leap. Either way, they made what they thought was an impossible change. Skim milk probably seemed watered down at first. Now that these people are used to skim, whole milk probably tastes too thick and rich. It's a small change, but when combined with other small dietary shifts, it all adds up to a healthier diet.

Take a moment to think about other changes you've faced in your life and how you adjusted. The strengths you relied on then may help you now. Use them.

Chapter 15
So I slipped up — what do I do?

OK, so you slipped up and fell off your eating plan. That happens. Everyone experiences challenges sooner or later. It doesn't do any good to get all bent out of shape about it. You can't change the past. What does help is analyzing what happened so you can try to avoid the situation again.

Even with a good plan and the best of intentions, you'll run into roadblocks now and then. How you respond to these obstacles can be the difference between success and failure.

Here's a look at some common problems that can cause a lapse in your diet and exercise plans and what you can do about them.

Plateaus

There's no greater reward for your effort than to step on the scale and see that you've lost weight. But what happens when the indicator on the scale doesn't change from week to week, even if you're eating a healthy, low-calorie diet and exercising regularly? Or you see results for the first few weeks, then hit a plateau? Days may go by, occasionally weeks, when your weight remains unchanged.

Before you get discouraged, understand that long-term results don't always show up right away. It's normal to hit plateaus. Some may even be due to your program. For example, exercise builds muscle. Muscle weighs more

than fat. You can have more muscle, less fat, look trimmer but not weigh less — but you've still made progress that the scale doesn't show.

Above all, when you hit a plateau, don't give up! Stick with the program. But make sure you're on track with weight-loss basics. Consider one of the strategies in the Action Guide (pages 180-207). Or try one of these tips:

+ Assess your food and activity records. **JOT IT** ▸ Make sure you haven't loosened the rules, letting yourself get by with larger portions or less exercise.

+ Focus on three- to four-week trends in weight loss instead of daily fluctuations. You may find that, although progress is not evident immediately, you're losing weight.

+ If you've hit a plateau, reassess your program. Is it possible that you've accomplished about as much as you can with the goals you've set? If so, you may need to adjust or change your program if you want to achieve more.

Lapse and relapse

A lapse occurs when you revert to old behaviors once or twice. It's temporary, common and a sign that you need to get back in control.

A relapse is more serious. After several lapses have occurred in a short span of time, you're at risk of completely reverting back to your old behavior. You panic, afraid that you'll undo all your good efforts. You may give up and say, "I guess I just can't do it."

Calm down. Take a deep breath. Remember that lapses are normal, temporary and can be anticipated. Consider these tips for getting back on track when you experience a lapse:

+ **Don't let negative thoughts take over.** Remember that mistakes happen and that each day is a chance to start anew.

+ **Clearly identify the problem, then create a list of possible solutions.** Pick a solution to try. If it works, then you've got a plan for preventing another lapse. If it doesn't work, try the next solution and go through the same process until you find one that works.

+ **Get support.** Talk to family, friends or a professional counselor.

+ **Work out your guilt and frustration with exercise.** Take a walk or go for a swim. Keep the exercise upbeat. Don't use exercise as punishment for a lapse.

+ **Recommit to your goals.** Review them and make sure they're still realistic.

What if you do relapse? Although relapses are disappointing, they can help you learn that your goals may be unrealistic, that certain situations create challenges for your program, or that certain strategies don't work.

Above all, realize that reverting to old behaviors doesn't mean that all hope is lost. It just means that you need to recharge your motivation, recommit to your program and return to healthy behaviors.

Stress

Everything is going along well until something happens that throws a wrench in your progress toward a healthy weight. When stressful situations occur, your natural response may be to abandon your program. You may turn to food for comfort. You may lose focus on your exercise routine.

Unfortunately, these solutions to stress can create a cycle of stress-related eating and a halt in exercise. See pages 136 and 141 in Chapter 14 for how to deal with stress.

Mood conditions

Clinical disorders such as depression and anxiety can put a halt to your weight program. There's a link between obesity and depression. So, if you show signs of a mood disorder, such as sleeping more than usual or feeling down a lot of the time, it's a good idea to seek professional help.

Talk to your doctor about your symptoms and treatment options. Generally, weight loss is easier once treatment

for the mood disorder is under way. Some medications for mood disorders can contribute to weight gain, so discuss alternatives with your doctor.

Breaking behavior chains

It's happened to everyone. You've had a healthy day — biked to work, eaten fresh fruit at breakfast and taken a 15-minute walk during your lunch break. Then a midafternoon craving sends you sprinting for the vending machine. Three minutes later, you're back at your desk with an extra-large candy bar in hand.

What happened? Maybe you were tired, or you didn't eat enough at lunch. Whatever the reason, you let a craving get the best of you. Now you feel guilty, frustrated and angry with yourself — feelings that may send you back to the vending machine. Where do you go from here?

Imagine this chain of events as a series of separate but interconnected behaviors. Try to separate this chain into discrete parts. Examining each link of the chain can lead to possible

Accentuate the positive

You start your day by stepping on the scale, and as the needle rises, you think, "I'll never be able to lose this extra weight." Maybe you decide to skip your morning walk because "it won't work anyway." At breakfast, you're so down that you top off your cereal with a doughnut and a glass of chocolate milk because, you think to yourself, "I've already blown my diet anyway. What does it matter?"

The scenario isn't uncommon, but it is unhealthy. Negative thoughts and attitudes can sabotage your weight-loss efforts. After all, why plan healthy meals and make a habit of exercising if defeat is certain?

The endless stream of thoughts running through your head every day is called self-talk. Often critical and negative, self-talk can discourage and weaken you to the point of despair.

You think: "I'm too fat." "I don't have any willpower." "The weight is coming off too slowly." "There must be something wrong with me."

On the other end of the spectrum is positive self-talk, which can be a powerful tool for building self-confidence, correcting bad habits, focusing attention, and solutions and help you control poor decision making that can lead to overeating.

Take the example of a woman who feels guilty after eating cookies but continues to eat more. Here's her chain of behavior:

1. Agrees to bring cookies instead of a salad to a friend's potluck dinner
2. Buys the cookies two days beforehand
3. Works late and misses her lunch
4. Arrives home very hungry
5. Thinks, "I'll eat one cookie, then go to the grocery store."

powering your exercise and eating routines. Positive self-talk is motivating and encouraging — the basis for many a successful life change. You're using positive self-talk when you bike up that steep hill, repeating all the while, "I can do it! I can do it!"

With a little practice, you can turn your negative self-talk into positive self-talk. Throughout the day, stop and evaluate what you're thinking. Question thoughts that you feel are upsetting, and then practice turning negative thoughts into positive statements. For instance, instead of saying, "It will never work," say, "I'll give it a try."

Some people find that they need outside help to change their negative thoughts into positive affirmations and to rid themselves of self-defeating attitudes and beliefs.

What's called cognitive behavioral therapy may help you do this. Cognitive behavioral therapy is based on the belief that much of what you are is what you think — that how you feel is a result of how you think about yourself and your life. If you're like many people, you allow your feelings to control your judgment ("I feel fat and ugly, so I must be fat and ugly"). You also magnify negative aspects of a situation while filtering out positive ones ("I've lost 5 pounds — but it's only 5 pounds, and I'll probably gain it back").

With cognitive behavioral therapy, a licensed therapist helps you replace these negative thoughts with more positive, realistic perceptions. Once you've learned new ways to view the events that make up your day, you're better able to cope with them.

6. Takes the box of cookies to the den
7. Eats cookies while watching television and reading her mail
8. Eats the cookies rapidly and without awareness
9. Feels guilty and like a failure
10. Eats more
11. Quits her weight program

At every link, she could have done something to break the chain of events. She could have agreed to bring a salad or a dessert she doesn't crave. She could have waited until the day of the party to buy the cookies. She could have planned a healthy evening meal in advance, so that after missing lunch, her eating wouldn't get out of control when she got home. She could have taken one or two cookies into the den, not the entire box. Finally, she could tell herself that this was a lapse and start again.

You can do the same with your behavior chains. Try interrupting a chain at the earliest link. If a midafternoon craving regularly strikes, you may break the chain by stocking your office desk with healthy snacks. Or maybe you can plan a healthy dinner before leaving for work. You'll face temptation. Have a plan for it.

Below are four different approaches to help break a behavior chain. Find one that works for you. If one approach isn't successful, try something else. Different approaches may work on different days.

ABC approach

Heading off problems before they develop can be effective in changing your behavior. This is sometimes called the ABC method: A stands for antecedent, B for behavior and C for

consequence. Most behaviors have a cause or antecedent. And behaviors lead to consequences.

Generally, people are more aware of the consequences of a behavior because these often demand their immediate attention. By addressing antecedents first, you may avert behaviors before they start and thus not have to deal with any consequences.

For example, keeping a tub of ice cream in the freezer (antecedent) may cause you to sneak spoonfuls throughout the day (behavior), ultimately causing you feelings of guilt and disrupting your weight program (consequence). Using the ABC approach, you might decide to keep ice cream out of your house entirely. This addresses the antecedent and helps you maintain your weight-control program.

Distraction approach

Imagine that ever since you were a child, you've enjoyed a bowl of ice cream before going to bed. So now, when you get ready for bed each night, the carton you've hidden in the back of

How to stay motivated

Staying motivated can keep you on track and help you avoid lapses and relapses. Motivation comes in many forms, but the best comes from within — your own personal reasons for wanting to lose weight. Use the process outlined on page 13 of Chapter 1 for identifying your own personal motivators. Here are some additional tips:

+ **Set goals.** Write them down and post them where you can see them. Focus on short-term goals and not just on a long-term weight-loss goal.

+ **Keep track of your progress.** Record exercise times, servings of food groups, pounds lost, milestones met and improvements in health. **JOT IT** ▸

+ **Put it in writing.** Make a contract with yourself and post it where you can see it.

+ **Create a support team.** Ask your family and friends to cheer you on (see page 151). Make time to exercise with them.

+ **Use rewards.** Reward yourself with something that matters to you every time you reach a goal.

+ **Recognize success.** As you lose weight and become more active, you'll likely feel better. Listen to your body to notice positve changes, and enjoy the success!

+ **Develop positive self-statements or affirmations.** Repeat them to yourself daily or type them and post them where you'll see them regularly. An example is, "I'm getting stronger and better every day," or that old standby, "Every day in every way, I'm getting better and better."

+ **Cut yourself some slack.** When it comes to your exercise program, remember that you're not in boot camp. It's OK to take a day off now and then when you need it. The more you make your weight program your own, the less likely you are to rebel against it.

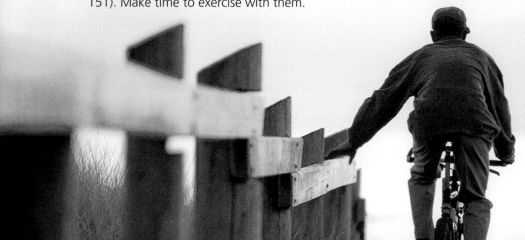

the freezer starts calling your name. Focus on turning your attention away from your craving. For instance, you might read, listen to music, write a letter or switch on the television.

Whatever your solution, the key is to find something that keeps your attention until the craving passes. Cravings are short-lived when your mind is occupied with something else.

Confrontation approach

This approach involves facing the negative consequences of your behavior head-on. For example, if you're craving ice cream, think about the unnecessary calories and fat you'll be consuming.

Think about how tired and sluggish you'll feel afterward. Think about how overeating will impact your health. Remind yourself that this isn't what you want to do with your life.

Give yourself a pat on the back for being able to say no to this craving this time. Yes, you can do it! And you will be able to do it again next time — and most times!

Shaping approach

Shaping encourages you to change your behavior gradually, one step at a time. For instance, instead of cutting ice cream out of your diet entirely, you eat a smaller bowl every night. Then you eliminate one evening snack completely — deciding, for example, to not eat ice cream on Mondays. In time, you'll be able to scale back to a small bowl of ice cream once a week. That's a nice compromise.

In some situations, making gradual changes over time can be less intimidating than is changing your life in a single day. As you succeed with step-by-step changes, your confidence will grow and will fuel further successes.

Adjusting your attitude

Maintaining a successful weight program requires more than adjusting your behaviors. The attitudes you have about yourself and about your body also affect your success. Following are five common problems that you may encounter, along with strategies for overcoming them.

Getting family and friends on board

It's difficult to lose weight alone, but it's even more challenging when those closest to you aren't supportive. Whether it's a partner who doesn't want to share your experience, a mother who insists that you eat her famous dessert, or friends who beg you to skip a work-out to go out for pizza, handling these relationships can make the road ahead difficult.

Help turn the tables in your favor with these suggestions:

- **Reach out.** Call on your weight-loss partners or a support group led by a health professional. They can help you counteract the temptations or negative messages you're getting from others.

- **Support yourself.** To remind yourself every day why you're changing your behaviors, post positive messages where you'll see them. Make a point of looking at them several times a day.

- **Provide reassurance.** It's not uncommon for a partner or companion to feel threatened as you lose weight and improve yourself and perhaps your appearance. Remind your loved one that while you're changing your lifestyle, you're not changing your feelings for him or her.

- **Ask for support.** Tell family and friends that you'd appreciate their help. Give them specific ways they can assist you.

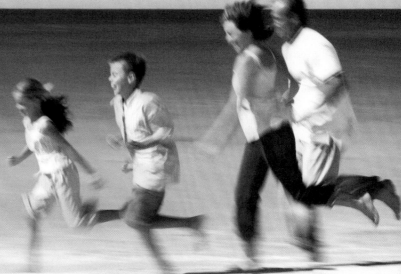

Finding activities to do as a family is great way to build healthy habits. Going to the beach, walks or hikes are just a few examples.

1. Negative self-talk

Self-talk — the internal dialog you have with yourself each day — influences your actions. When that self-talk is negative, it can weaken your self-esteem and stall your progress. After all, if you convince yourself that you'll never lose weight, it seems reasonable to say to yourself, "Why even try in the first place?"

Remove yourself from this self-defeating behavior by replacing negative self-talk with positive self-talk.

2. Negative attitude

Negative attitudes and beliefs can be as destructive as negative self-talk. For instance, you may believe that you can't go to the gym because people will stare and make fun of your body. Or maybe you credit a special diet for your initial success instead of your own abilities and hard work. Such perceptions can sabotage your ability to lose weight.

Fight back by identifying your negative attitudes. Write them down and think of alternative attitudes to counteract them. Consider these examples:

+ **Negative attitude** — "Exercise is painful and boring."

+ **New attitude** — "I like being physically active. I'll call a friend to go walking and enjoy the beautiful day."

+ **Negative attitude** — "I'm only losing weight because this program works. Once it's over, I'll regain the weight."

+ **New attitude** — "I'm making this happen by making positive choices. My success will continue even when my program ends because I'm committed to changing my lifestyle for a lifetime."

3. Unrealistic dreams

Sometimes, you may imagine that losing weight will cure all your problems. But you know this is an unrealistic expectation.

Be realistic about what weight loss will do for you. Yes, you'll probably be healthier and you'll likely have more energy and higher self-esteem. But losing weight doesn't guarantee a better social life or more satisfying job.

Your life will likely change with weight loss, but slowly — and maybe not in the ways that you imagine. Try to counteract unrealistic dreaming with these strategies:

+ **Set realistic expectations.** Recognize your unrealistic dreams, then counter them with more-rational goals.

+ **Set short-term, realistic goals.** Instead of focusing on how happy you'll be after reaching your ultimate weight goal, focus on small, achievable goals toward which you can make progress — ones that you are able to measure daily or weekly. This gives you the opportunity to celebrate successes every week.

+ **Celebrate changed behaviors.** Don't just reward yourself for pounds lost. You're working hard, and there are other achievements to be excited about.

4. Inflexibility

Words such as *always, must* and *never* add undue pressure to your program. For instance, you decide that you'll "never eat chocolate again." Or you demand, "I must walk two miles every single day."

Why be so tough on yourself? After all, to *never* or *always* do anything is a lot to ask and may be a path to guilt-ridden lapses.

This urgency doesn't allow you to be flexible, and everyone makes mistakes. Besides, if you beat yourself up over one momentary slip, it's easy to overlook the progress you're making. Denying yourself something, such as chocolate, may actually fuel a craving. When you finally break down, you may be as apt to buy two candy bars as you are one.

Once you've broken your rule, you may allow yourself to have chocolate ice cream before dinner or chocolate cake before bed. Suddenly, your eat-no-chocolate rule has made you feel like a failure.

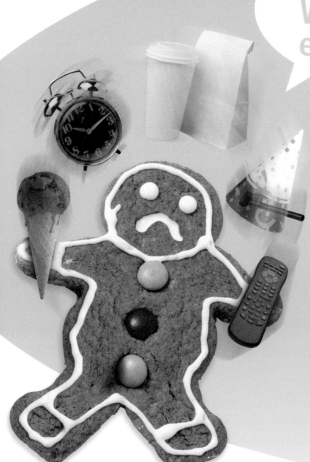

What are your eating triggers?

One way to prevent a recurrence of overeating is to identify situations that cause you trouble. Consider what your eating triggers might be, and plot strategies to overcome them.

Time of day

Are there certain times of the day when you're more susceptible to overeating? Maybe you do well in the mornings and afternoons but have a tough time with food cravings in the evenings. Or, perhaps, in that lull between lunch and dinner, you get a strong, uncontrollable urge to snack.

Emotions

Food is a common response to a negative mood. Do you find that certain feelings

The sensible approach is to plan for a treat now and then but do so in appropriate situations — for example, when you're out to dinner with friends but not when you're alone or feeling sad.

5. All-or-nothing thinking

All-or-nothing thinking causes you to see a situation as either all good or all bad. For instance, you may think, "If I exceed my calorie count today, I'm back to being overweight," or "If I skip the treadmill, I've blown the program." In short, what you feel is, "If I'm not perfect, I'm a failure."

Few things about weight loss are all or nothing. One setback doesn't mean you're a failure. If you let yourself cause you to snack mindlessly? Do you tend to eat when you're bored, lonely, depressed, stessed or anxious?

Activities

Do you find that you eat more when doing certain activities? Is reading the newspaper or sitting at the computer without food in hand a problem for you? Do you find yourself constantly snacking while watching television or preparing a meal? Is food how you deal with activities that you don't enjoy, such as paying bills or doing homework?

Social situations

Have you noticed that you eat more when you're around certain people? Maybe it's a good friend who likes to go out to eat or frequently invites you over for coffee and a "little snack." Maybe it's when your partner gets the nibbles, and you eat, too.

Foods

Do you find that you just can't eat some foods in moderation, such as ice cream, chocolate, or chips and salsa? Does the smell of pancakes and sausage or fresh cookies from the oven cause you to completely forget about your eating plan?

Physical factors

Does how you feel cause you to overeat? If you skip breakfast, do hunger pangs cause you to lose control of your eating. When you're fatigued, do you turn to junk food for energy? Do you use food to help distract you from chronic pain?

believe this, you're likely to suffer guilt and depression and take a serious blow to your self-esteem. And as the problem snowballs, you may be tempted to handle those feelings by giving up.

Counteract all-or-nothing thinking with moderation. Tell yourself, for instance, that there are no "good" and "bad" foods, and that it's OK to have dessert once in a while.

Or, instead of calling yourself a failure when you eat more than you planned or miss an exercise session, remind yourself that you can get back on track tomorrow. Be realistic in your assessment of your behaviors. Slip-ups happen, but you can overcome them.

Chapter 16
Making meals easy

When you eat at home, you consume fewer calories. But homemade meals take time, and it seems we never have enough of that — especially when it comes to meals. In order to have great, tasty, healthy meals, you need a good process for planning them. This chapter can help.

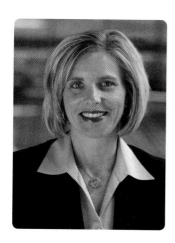

Kris Schmitz
Clinical Nutrition

When I work with people who are motivated to change how they eat, among the first things we discuss are ways to implement these changes. Here are a few ideas I've found beneficial:

+ Intentionally plan for leftovers. By making enough for two meals at once, you'll save time. Leftovers make a great lunch brought from home.
+ Incorporate balance each time you eat: lean protein/low-fat dairy, whole grains, fruits and vegetables, and moderate fat.
+ Keep a running grocery list in the kitchen so items can be added as needed.
+ Create the list in order of where foods are located in your favorite store, to reduce shopping time.
+ Enlist others at home to plan menus, prepare food and shop with you. To save time when shopping, assign each person a different section of the store to pick up items on the list. Limit the items you purchase that are not on your list.
+ Don't forget to incorporate sale and seasonal items to save money and maximize flavor.
+ Keep a coupon file to save you money.
+ Create a binder or card file of favorite recipes that you can refer to over time if you need inspiration.

Start with small steps. If you rarely eat at home, start with one or two meals a week and gradually add more. Over time, you'll notice that you'll be eating mindfully, which leads to healthier choices. And remember — be flexible, have fun and engage others!

It starts with shopping

You can't eat what you don't have, and that goes for foods that can help your weight-loss plans (and for those that can sabatoge your efforts). Follow these strategies to ensure that you have the right foods on hand.

Step 1: Plan ahead

Decide how many major meals you'll be shopping for. Then, consider the food items you'll need for breakfasts, lunches and snacks. Take an inventory of your staples, such as low-fat milk, fresh fruits and whole grains. See page 159 for ideas. **JOT IT** ▸

Step 2: Make a list

A list makes your shopping trip more efficient and helps you avoid impulse purchases. But don't let your list prevent you from looking for or trying new healthy foods.

When making your list, use your weight-loss menus as your guide. Make sure your list includes healthy and convenient snack foods.

Step 3: Shop the perimeter of the store for fresh foods

Chances are that the fresh produce, dairy case, and meat and seafood sections of your grocery store are all located on the perimeter. That's where to focus your shopping when using the Mayo Clinic Healthy Weight Pyramid. Fresh foods are generally better than ready-to-eat foods because you can control any ingredients that you add.

Step 4: Don't shop when hungry

It's harder to resist buying high-fat, high-calorie snack items when you're hungry. So set yourself up for success and shop after you've eaten a good meal. If you do find yourself shopping on an empty stomach, drink some water or buy a piece of fruit to munch on.

Step 5: Read nutrition labels

Check nutrition labels for serving size, calories, fat, cholesterol and sodium. Remember, even low-fat and fat-free foods can pack a lot of calories. Compare similar products so that you can choose the healthiest options.

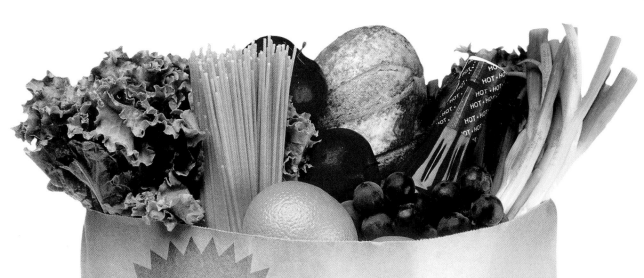

STOCK UP!
on these healthy items

Healthy meals can come together in minutes — if you have what you need. Plan shopping lists so that you keep the following items on hand:

FRUITS AND VEGETABLES

+ Fresh fruits
+ Canned fruits (packed in their own juice or water)
+ Frozen fruits
+ Fresh vegetables
+ Pre-cut fresh vegetables
+ Frozen vegetables (no sauce)
+ Salad in a bag
+ Fat-free tomato sauce
+ 100% fruit juice (but limit juice intake to 4 ounces a day)

WHOLE GRAINS

+ Whole-grain breakfast cereal
+ Rice (brown, wild, blends)
+ Oatmeal
+ Whole-grain bread
+ Whole-grain pita bread
+ Whole-grain pasta

PROTEIN

+ Low-fat refried beans
+ Black, kidney or navy beans
+ Low-sodium water-packed tuna
+ Other fish with omega-3s
+ Skinless white meat poultry
+ Soy cheese
+ Tofu

DAIRY

+ Low-fat or fat-free yogurt
+ Low-fat or fat-free cheese
+ Fat-free or 1% milk

How to read the nutrition label

Keep these simple tips in mind:

❶ **Check the serving size**
How many servings are in the container?

❷ **Check the calories in one serving**

❸ **Check the % Daily Value***
5% or less is low
20% or more is high

*Percent Daily Value (DV) in one serving is based on a 2,000-calorie diet for adults. For example, the recommended goal for dietary fiber is 25 grams, so 1 gram is 4% DV. Your DV may be higher or lower, depending on your calorie needs.

**Keep intake of saturated fat and trans fat as low as possible. All fats are high in calories.

Adapted from FDA, Center for Food Safety and Applied Nutrition, 2006

Nutrition Facts

Serving Size 16 Crackers (31 g)
Servings Per Container About 9

Amount Per Serving

Calories 150 — Calories from Fat 50

% Daily Value*

Total Fat 6 g**	**9%**
Saturated Fat 1 g	**6%**
Trans Fat 1 g	
Polyunsaturated Fat 2 g	
Monounsaturated Fat 2 g	
Cholesterol 0 mg	**0%**
Sodium 270 mg	**11%**
Total Carbohydrate 21 g	**7%**
Dietary Fiber 1 g	**4%**
Sugars 3 g	
Protein 8 g	

Vitamin A 4%	Vitamin C 2%
Calcium 20%	Iron 4%

Limit nutrients
shown in orange

Get enough
of nutrients
shown in green

Quick & healthy menu ideas

Sautéed vegetables

Sauté cherry tomatoes, asparagus, bell peppers, broccoli, onion and other vegetables. Toss with cooked whole-wheat pasta and a splash of olive oil. Top with grated Parmesan cheese.

Vegetables = multiple servings

⅓ cup pasta = 1 Carbohydrate

1 teaspoon oil = 1 Fat

Summer salad

Top bed of crisp romaine lettuce with a thinly sliced fresh (or canned in juice) whole pear. Sprinkle with four chopped pecans. Add a few shavings of Parmesan cheese. Drizzle with low-fat French dressing.

Lettuce = 1 Vegetable

Pear = 1 Fruit

Pecans & dressing = 2 Fat (Parmesan not enough to count)

Nibbler platter

Arrange baby carrots, celery sticks, red bell pepper chunks, zucchini rounds, sliced apple and whole-wheat crackers on a platter. Use these items to pick up and eat ½ cup (3 ounces) tuna.

Vegetables = multiple servings

Apple = 1 Fruit

8 crackers = 1 Carbohydrate

Tuna = 1 Protein/Dairy

Pocket salad

Stuff half of a 6-inch whole-wheat pita with chopped vegetables (lettuce, carrot, zucchini, cucumbers). Top with favorite low-fat dressing.

Vegetables = multiple servings

Pita = 1 Carbohydrate

Dressing = 1 Fat

Stir-fry

Cook quick brown rice while also stir-frying a bag of mixed, ready-to-eat vegetables in a little peanut oil. Toss vegetables with a teaspoon of Thai peanut sauce to spice up the flavor.

Vegetables = multiple servings

⅓ cup rice = 1 Carbohydrate

Using only a small amount of oil and sauce (1 teaspoon each) will count as about 1 fat.

Quick soup

Bring to boil 1 quart reduced-sodium chicken broth. Cook any amount of fresh or leftover vegetables (for example, carrots, onions, green beans, mushrooms, rutabagas, tomatoes or zucchini) until vegetables are tender. Serve with 8 whole-wheat crackers or slice of whole-wheat toast.

Vegetables = multiple servings

Crackers or toast = 1 Carbohydrate

Refreshing fruit snacks

Freeze any of the following fresh fruit: 1 cup or about 30 grapes, 1 small banana, 1½ cups hulled strawberries, 1 large peeled and sliced kiwi fruit, ½ cup or 2 rings pineapple, ¾ cup peaches, ½ cup mango. Serve when ready.

Amounts shown = 1 Fruit

Fiesta wrap

Rinse canned black beans in strainer. Move beans to microwave-safe dish and microwave until hot. Wrap shredded lettuce, chopped onion and tomato, a spoonful of beans and salsa in 6-inch whole-wheat tortilla.

Vegetables = 1 serving

1 tortilla = 1 Carbohydrate

½ cup beans = 1 Protein/Dairy

Healthy cooking

Healthy cooking doesn't mean you have to become a gourmet chef or invest in special cookware. Simply use standard cooking methods to prepare foods in healthy ways. You can also adapt familiar recipes by substituting other ingredients for fat, sugar and salt (see page 164).

Use these methods

These methods best capture the flavor and retain the nutrients in your food without adding too much fat or salt.

+ **Baking.** Besides breads and desserts, you can bake seafood, poultry, lean meat, and vegetable and fruit pieces of the same size. Place food in a pan or dish (covered or uncovered) and bake. You may need to baste the food with broth, low-fat marinade or juice to keep the food from drying out.

+ **Braising.** Braising involves browning the meat or poultry first in a pan on top of the stove, and then slowly cooking it covered with a small amount of liquid, such as water or broth. In some recipes, the cooking liquid is used afterward to form a flavorful, nutrient-rich sauce.

+ **Grilling and broiling.** Both grilling and broiling expose fairly thin pieces of food to direct heat and allow fat to drip away from the food. If you're grilling outdoors, place smaller items, such as chopped vegetables, in a long-handled grill basket or on foil to prevent pieces from slipping through the rack. To broil indoors, place food on a broiler rack below a heat element.

+ **Poaching.** To poach foods, in a covered pan gently simmer ingredients in water or a flavorful liquid, such as broth, vinegar or juice, until cooked through and tender. For stove-top poaching, choose an appropriate-sized covered pan and use a minimum amount of liquid.

+ **Roasting.** Roasting uses an oven's dry heat at high temperatures to cook the food on a baking sheet or in a roasting pan. For poultry, seafood and meat, place a rack inside the roasting pan so that the fat can drip away during cooking.

+ **Sautéing.** Sautéing quickly cooks small or thin pieces of food. If you choose a good-quality nonstick pan, you can cook food without using fat. Depending on the recipe, use low-sodium broth, cooking spray, water or wine in place of oil or butter.

+ **Steaming.** One of the simplest cooking techniques to master is steaming food in a perforated basket suspended above simmering liquid. If you use a flavorful liquid or add herbs to the water, you'll flavor the food as it cooks.

+ **Stir-frying.** Stir-frying quickly cooks small, uniform-sized pieces of food while they're rapidly stirred in a wok or large nonstick frying pan. You need only a small amount of oil or cooking spray for this cooking method.

Find new ways to add flavor

Instead of salt or butter, you can enhance foods with a variety of herbs, spices and low-fat condiments. Be creative.

Poach fish in low-fat broth or wine and fresh herbs. Top a broiled chicken breast with fresh salsa. Make meats more flavorful with low-fat marinades or spices — bay leaf, chili powder, dry mustard, garlic, ginger, green pepper, sage, marjoram, onion, oregano, pepper or thyme.

To bring out the sweetness in baked goods, use a bit more vanilla, cinnamon or nutmeg.

Adapting recipes

If the recipe calls for	Try substituting
Butter Margarine Shortening Oil	✚ For sandwiches, substitute tomato slices, catsup or mustard. ✚ For stove-top cooking, sauté food in broth or small amounts of healthy oil like olive, canola or peanut or use non-stick spray. ✚ In marinades, substitute diluted fruit juice, wine or balsamic vinegar. ✚ In cakes or bars, replace half the fat or oil with the same amount of applesauce, prune puree or commercial fat substitute. ✚ To avoid dense, soggy or flat baked goods, don't substitute oil for butter or shortening, or substitute diet, whipped or tub-style margarine for regular margarine.
Meat	Keep it lean. In soup, chili or stir-fry, replace most of the meat with beans or vegetables. As an entrée, keep it to no more than the size of a deck of cards — load up on vegetables.
Whole milk (regular or evaporated)	Fat-free or 1% milk, or evaporated skim milk
Whole egg (yolk and white)	¼ cup egg substitute or 2 egg whites for breakfast or in baked goods
Sour cream Cream cheese	Fat-free, low-fat or light varieties in dips, spreads, salad dressings and toppings. Fat-free, low-fat and light varieties do not work well for baking.
Sugar	In most baked goods, you can reduce the amount of sugar by one-half without affecting texture or taste, but use no less than ¼ cup of sugar for every cup of flour to keep items moist.
White flour	Replace half or more of white flour with whole grain pastry or regular flour.
Salt	✚ Use herbs (1 tbsp. fresh = 1 tsp. dried = ¼ tsp. powder). Add towards the end of cooking and use sparingly — you can always add more. ✚ Salt is required when baking yeast-leavened items. Otherwise you may reduce salt by half in cookies and bars. Not needed when boiling pasta.

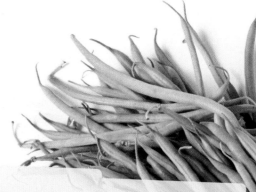

Sample menus

These 1,200-calorie menus give you generous servings of vegetables and fruits, four servings of carbohydrates, and three servings each of protein/dairy and fats. If your daily calorie goal is higher, you'll need to adjust the menus accordingly.

Breakfast

+ **Fruit yogurt parfait** (1 cup fat-free yogurt mixed with 1 serving fruit)

Lunch

+ **1 serving tuna and pasta salad** (Combine 1 can water-packed tuna, 4 cups cooked shell pasta, 2 cups diced carrots and zucchini, and 4 tablespoons low-calorie mayonnaise — serves 4)
+ **1 small orange**

Dinner

+ **⅓ 12-inch crust cheese pizza**
+ **Green salad** (2 cups lettuce with ½ cup sliced tomatoes, red onions and mushrooms)
+ **2 tablespoons fat-free salad dressing**

Snack

+ **1 small apple, sliced**

Include a calorie-free beverage with each meal.

Breakfast

+ **Omelet** (Mix ½ cup egg substitute with ½ cup diced onions, tomatoes, green peppers and mushrooms. Cook until set.)
+ **1 slice whole-grain toast**
+ **1 teaspoon trans fat-free margarine**
+ **1 medium orange**

Lunch

+ **Hummus pita** (Mash ⅓ cup garbanzos with 1 teaspoon extra-virgin olive oil. Add garlic, cumin, lemon and parsley to taste. Place in whole-grain pita.)
+ **Cucumber and tomato salad** (Mix 1 cup sliced cucumber and 8 cherry tomatoes, halved. Add herb-flavored vinegar.)
+ **1 cup grapes**

Dinner

+ **3 ounces grilled perch or other fish**
+ **½ cup cooked lemon-peppered, whole-grain pasta**
+ **⅔ cup green beans**
+ **1 cup berries**

Snack

+ **9 large olives**

Include a calorie-free beverage with each meal.

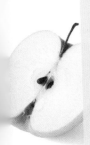

Chapter 17
Sticking to the diet when eating out

Eating out is convenient, efficient, sometimes essential —
and let's face it, *fun*. It's also associated with weight gain.
But by adopting a few healthy habits, you can enjoy eating
out without packing on extra pounds.

You *can* eat away from home without sabotaging your weight-loss plan. You just need to be menu-savvy about making decisions. You also need to be mindful of two common dining-out challenges: the urge to order more food than you need and the impulse to eat every bit of food on your plate — even when the portion sizes are way too large for one meal.

Maneuvering the menu

When ordering food at a restaurant, do you know which items may be loaded with fat and calories? Unlike when you're grocery shopping, the foods in a restaurant may not have nutrition labels listing their fat and calorie content.

Hidden calories refer to the extra calories in many dishes that come from ingredients you may be unaware of. That's why they're such a problem for people grappling with weight control. Ingredients often are added to enhance the flavor, color or texture of food — for example, seasonings, sauces, cheesy toppings or dressings. And sometimes they're part of the

process used to prepare the dish — for example, oil or butter for cooking. These calories add up.

Use these tips to steer clear of hidden fat and calories in restaurant food:

+ **Appetizers.** If you're having an appetizer, choose one that contains primarily vegetables, fruit or fish. Tomato juice, fresh fruit compote and shrimp cocktail served with lemon are healthy appetizers. Avoid fried or breaded appetizers, which are generally high in calories.

+ **Soup.** The best choices are broth-based or tomato-based soups. Creamed soups, chowders and puréed soups can contain heavy cream or egg yolks.

+ **Bread.** Muffins, garlic toast and croissants have more fat and calories than do whole-grain bread, breadsticks and crackers. Skip the temptation by asking the server not to bring the breadbasket.

+ **Salad.** Your best choice is a lettuce or spinach salad with a low-fat

Clues on the Menu

Avoid these terms:

A la king

Au gratin

Basted

Breaded

Broasted

Buttered

Creamed

Fricasseed

Fried

Hollandaise sauce

Sautéed or stir-fried in heavy oil

Look for these terms:

Baked

Broiled, without added butter

Grilled

Poached

Roasted

Sautéed or stir-fried in a small amount of oil, broth or water

Steamed

dressing on the side. Limit all of the high-calorie add-ons, such as cheese and croutons.

Chef salad and taco salad are usually high in fat and calories because of the meat, cheese and other extras — such as the taco salad's deep-fried shell.

+ **Side dish.** Choose steamed vegetables, rice, fresh fruits, a baked potato or boiled new potatoes instead of higher calorie options, such as french fries, potato chips and mayonnaise-based salads.

+ **Entrees.** You may want to skip pasta dishes with meat or cheese or dishes with creamy sauces. The names of certain dishes indicate that they're high in fat, such as prime rib, veal parmigiana, stuffed shrimp, fried chicken, fried rice and fettuccine Alfredo. Many other cooking terms also give you a basic idea of a food's nutritional makeup.

+ **Dessert.** Finish your main meal before ordering dessert. By the time you're done, you may not even want dessert. If you do order dessert, consider splitting it with one of your companions. Some healthy dessert options include fresh fruit, sorbet or sherbet.

Assessing the salad bar

When dining out, you may think that eating at the salad bar is a healthy alternative to ordering from the menu. But unless you make careful choices, you could end up with a plate filled with calories and fat.

Before you order, walk through the salad bar to see if it has ingredients you like to make a tasty yet healthy salad. Some salad bars look more like a delicatessen, with a lot of rich, high-fat options. Remember that just because a food is located in the salad bar doesn't mean that it's healthy.

+ **Go green.** Lettuce or fresh spinach is generally the foundation of a healthy salad. Do the greens look fresh and plentiful?

+ **Survey the fresh fruits and vegetables.** In addition to greens, you want to pile on fresh vegetables and fruits, such as tomatoes, mushrooms, carrots, broccoli, cauliflower, cucumbers, beets, radishes, bell peppers, pineapple, cantaloupe, watermelon, grapes and strawberries. Is there a good offering of these items?

+ **Acknowledge the extras.** Many people go wrong at salad bars by including too many high-fat ingredients. These include items such as cheese, chopped eggs, bacon bits and buttery croutons, or other types of salads such as pasta salad or potato salad.

When you go through the salad bar, take only very small amounts of these items or avoid them altogether.

+ **Don't forget the dressings.** Look for fat-free or low-fat, low-calorie dressings, such as low-fat Italian or reduced-calorie French. Other options include vinegars. You can also add flavor to your salad with herbs and peppers. Check to see if any seasonings are available.

YOUR GUIDE TO HEALTHY ETHNIC CUISINE

These suggestions will help you savor the exotic, while keeping calories, fat, cholesterol and sodium under control.

 ## Chinese

✔ **Look for:** Stir-fried (ask to have it prepared in little or no oil) or steamed dishes with lots of vegetables, steamed rice, poached fish, and hot and sour soups.

✘ **Avoid:** Fatty spareribs, fried wontons, egg rolls, shrimp toast and fried rice. To limit sodium, ask that your food be prepared without salt or monosodium glutamate (MSG). Request soy sauce (high in sodium) and other sauces on the side.

French

✔ **Look for:** Steamed shellfish, roasted poultry, salad with dressing on the side, and sauces with a wine or tomato base, such as bordelaise or à la Provençal.

✘ **Avoid:** French onion soup (high in sodium; high in fat if it has cheese), high-fat sauces (béchamel, hollandaise and béarnaise), croissants and pâté.

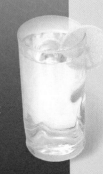

Water anyone?

Soft drinks and alcohol-containing beverages can quickly add calories to any restaurant experience. Focus on no- or low-calorie drink options.

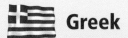 # Greek

✔ **Look for:** Plaki (fish cooked with toma-toes, onions and garlic), chicken kebabs (chicken broiled on a spit with tomatoes, onions and peppers), or a Greek salad.

✗ **Avoid:** Dishes with large amounts of butter or oil, such as baba ghanouj (eggplant appetizer) and baklava (dessert made with phyllo dough, butter, nuts and honey). To limit sodium, avoid olives, anchovies and feta cheese.

 # Japanese

✔ **Look for:** Steamed rice, soba or udon noodles, yakisoba (stir-fried noodles), yakitori (chicken teriyaki), shumai (steamed dumplings), tofu, sukiyaki, kayaku gohan (vegetables and rice).

✗ **Avoid:** Shrimp or vegetable tempura, chicken katsu, tonkatsu (fried pork), shrimp agemono, fried tofu (bean curd).

 # Italian

✔ **Look for:** Marinara (tomatoes with garlic and onions), Marsala (based in wine), clam sauce and pasta primavera with fresh vegetables and a small amount of oil. Simply prepared fish and chicken dishes also are good choices.

✗ **Avoid:** Pasta stuffed with cheese or fatty meat and dishes with cream or butter sauces. Veal scaloppine and parmigiana (cooked with Parmesan cheese) contain added fat.

 # Mexican

✔ **Look for:** Grilled fish, shrimp and chicken with salsa made of tomato, chilies and onion. Order corn tortillas (they're lower in fat and calories than are flour tortillas) as long as they aren't deep-fried. For a side dish, order rice or beans (black, pinto, refried). Make sure your side dishes aren't cooked with fat or lard — ask your server about this.

✗ **Avoid:** Dishes with large amounts of cheese, sour cream and guacamole. Chips also can add a lot of fat and calories.

Chapter 18
Burning even more calories

If you want to burn calories, move. If you want to burn even more calories, move more. It's pretty much that simple. Chapter 9 touched on some of the basics of burning calories through increased physical activity. Here, we go into a little more depth.

The cool thing about burning calories is that the possibilities are almost endless. You don't even have to sweat.

You can go long — as in duration — but with low intensity, just moving a lot throughout the day. Or if a bit of perspiration doesn't turn you off, you can burn a lot of calories with short, high-intensity activity — if you can handle it (see page 175).

A balanced program includes aerobic activities to help burn calories, and strength training, core stability exercises and stretching to make your activities safe and more effective.

Be flexible in your planning. Create a routine that fits your schedule and interests. Maybe you can walk for an hour on most days and do strength exercises for 20 minutes three times a week. Do what works for you.

Once you're in the habit, exercising regularly will feel comfortable. You may look forward to the break from other obligations. And remember, you don't have to do your daily exercises all at one time.

Key points

Whether you go with low-intensity physical activity or full-blown exercise, remember these key points:

+ Start with activities that match your current fitness level and build at a reasonable pace to a higher level.
+ In building up, first increase the frequency of your exercise (number of days a week), then as you become more fit, the duration (length of each activity session), and finally the intensity (how hard you're working).
+ Make it fun, or you won't stick with your program.
+ Keep activity in balance with the rest of your life (but make it an important part of that balance).

Schedule time for rest in your routine. Your body needs to recover between exercise sessions. Alternate between low-intensity and higher intensity exercise from day to day.

The following pages give you a little more depth on aerobics, strength training, core training and stretching.

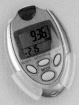

Getting started with walking

A simple walking program, such as the example below, may be the best aerobic activity to start with, especially if you haven't been particularly active. Start with slow, short walks and gradually increase your frequency, time and intensity.

Once you can walk a distance without much strain, you can vary the intensity by walking hills, increasing your pace or swinging your arms more. Your ultimate goal is to be active about an hour a day.

Adapt this program to suit your needs. If it's too easy, pick it up a bit. If it's too hard, back off. Variety may help — pick two days out of the week for longer walks, and have the rest be shorter. If you can't start out walking 15 minutes, start with what you can do and work up.

Week	Minutes/day	Comments
1	15	4 days this week
2	20	5 days this week
3	25	Begin 7 days a week
4	30	
5	35	
6	40	Increase intensity
7	45	
8	50	
9	55	
10	60	Increase intensity

Aerobics

Aerobic means "with oxygen." Aerobic activities are done at an intensity that you can keep up for a moderately long time without getting winded. This allows you to burn a lot of calories, helping with weight loss.

Include three elements in your aerobic workout:

+ **Warm-up.** Before each session, warm up for five to 10 minutes to gradually rev up your cardiovascular system and increase blood flow to your muscles. Try a low-intensity version of your planned activity. For example, if you plan to walk, warm up by walking slowly. Then stretch.

+ **Conditioning.** Do your aerobic activity.

+ **Cool-down.** After each session, cool down for five to 10 minutes. Stretch your calf muscles, upper thighs, hamstrings, lower back and chest. This after-workout stretch allows your heart rate and muscles to return to normal.

Speed calorie burn with higher intensity

If you're interested in burning even more calories, and are physically capable of the effort, higher intensity exercise may help.

When you exercise, the increase in activity boosts the number of calories you burn, not just during the activity but for a while afterward as well. With low-intensity activities, the afterburn tails off fairly quickly. But with higher intensity activities, the afterburn is longer.

Intervals are one example of a higher intensity activity. They involve repeated bursts of relatively intense activity separated by short recovery periods, such as cycling fairly hard for several minutes, then pedaling casually for a minute or two to recover, and repeating that several times. Intervals can also be part of a walking program, by walking fast for a while, then slower, and repeating.

Afterburn also can be extended without throwing in the short bursts, simply by increasing the intensity of activity. For example, you could walk more briskly throughout your normal walk.

Attempt intense activity only after you've built a foundation of fitness through less intense activity (remember, — frequency first, then duration, then intensity). And check with your doctor if you're uncertain about your health.

WARNING SIGNS: WHEN TO STOP

Moderate activity should cause you to breathe faster and feel like you're working. But if you experience any of these signs or symptoms during exercise, stop immediately and seek medical attention:

- Chest pain or tightness
- Dizziness or faintness
- Pain in an arm or your jaw
- Severe shortness of breath
- Excessive fatigue

- Bursts of very rapid or slow heart rate
- An irregular heartbeat
- Severe joint or muscle pain
- Joint swelling

Strength training

Strength training, also referred to as resistance training or weightlifting, builds the strength and endurance of your muscles. Strength training reduces body fat and increases lean muscle mass.

Increased lean muscle mass will provide you with a bigger "engine" to burn calories. Because muscle tissue burns more calories than does fat tissue, the more muscle mass you have, the more calories you burn, even at rest.

Strength training involves working your muscles against some form of resistance. Strength training is typically done with free weights, weight machines or resistance bands.

You can also exercise using the weight of your own body as the resistance with exercises such as push-ups, lunges and standing squats.

Regardless of the method you choose, begin strength training slowly. If you start with too much resistance or too many repetitions, you may damage muscles and joints. A single set of 12 repetitions (reps) can build muscle just as effectively as doing multiple sets. Start with a weight you can lift comfortably eight times and build up to 12 repetitions.

The weight should be heavy enough so that the last three to four repetitions are difficult to complete. After you can easily do 12 repetitions, increase the weight by up to 10 percent.

Before each session, take a five- to 10-minute walk to warm up your muscles. You can work your whole body during each session, or you can focus on your upper body during one session and your lower body during the next. To allow time for your muscles to recover, take at least one day off before working the same muscle group again.

If you're new to strength training, consider finding a certified professional, often found at fitness centers, to teach you the proper technique. Or look for a class offered through a community education program.

Here are strength-training guidelines:

+ **Complete all movements slowly and with control.** If you're unable to maintain good form, decrease the weight or number of reps.

+ **Breathe normally and freely, exhaling as you lift a weight and inhaling as you lower it.**

+ **Stop if you feel pain.**

+ **Stretch your muscles before and after working out.** When stretching beforehand, warm up first.

+ **Work at an intensity that you feel is somewhat hard.** You should feel a strain (not pain).

+ **Listen to your body.** Mild muscle soreness for a few days after starting strength training is normal, but sharp pain and sore or swollen joints can mean you've overdone it.

+ **Be consistent.** Three workouts a week, typically lasting 20 to 30 minutes each, will build muscle. Two will maintain strength.

Core stability

Your core — the area around your trunk and pelvis — is where all movement in your body originates. It's also where your center of gravity is located. A strong core provides a more stable platform for movement and helps you with other physical activities.

When you have good core stability, the muscles in your pelvis, lower back, hips and abdomen work in harmony and provide support to your spine. A weak core can make you susceptible to poor posture, lower back pain and muscle injuries.

Core strengthening requires the regular and proper exercise of your body's core muscles. Abdominal crunches are a form of core exercise. You can have fun doing some core exercises using a fitness ball. Balancing on these oversized, inflated balls requires that you focus on using your core muscles for support.

Do core exercises at least three times a week. Breathe steadily and slowly, and take a break when you need one. For optimal results, get help from a trained professional when you begin — body position and alignment are crucial when performing core-strengthening exercises.

Stretching and flexibility

Most aerobic and strength training programs cause your muscles to tighten. Stretching can increase flexibility and range of motion, helping you in your day-to-day activities and in the other components of your exercise program. When stretching:

+ **Target major muscle groups.** Focus on your calves, thighs, hips, lower back, neck and shoulders. Also stretch muscles and joints that you routinely use at work or play.

+ **Warm up first.** Stretching muscles when they're cold increases your risk of injury, including pulled muscles. Warm up by walking while gently pumping your arms, or do a favorite exercise at low intensity for five minutes. If you only have time to stretch once, do it after you exercise — when your muscles are warm.

+ **Hold each stretch for at least 30 seconds.** It takes time to lengthen tissues safely. Hold your stretches for up to 60 seconds for a really tight muscle or problem area. Then repeat the stretch on the other side. For most muscle groups, a single stretch is usually sufficient.

+ **Don't bounce.** Bouncing as you stretch can cause small tears in the muscle. These tears leave scar tissue as the muscle heals, which tightens the muscle even further — making you less flexible and more prone to pain.

+ **Focus on a pain-free stretch.** Expect to feel tension while you're stretching. If it hurts, you've gone too far. Back off to the point where you don't feel pain, then hold the stretch.

+ **Relax and breathe freely.** Don't hold your breath.

As a general rule, stretch whenever you exercise. If you're particularly tight, you might want to stretch every day or even twice a day.

You may want to sign up for a class on yoga or tai chi, which can promote flexibility. Plus, you may stick with a program better if you're in a class.

Calories burned in 1 hour

Calorie expenditure for a variety of activities varies widely depending on the type of exercise, intensity level and individual. If you weigh less than 160 pounds, your calories burned would be somewhat less than shown, and if you weigh more than 240 pounds, calories burned would be somewhat more.

Activity (one-hour duration)	WEIGHT OF PERSON AND CALORIES BURNED		
	160 POUNDS (73 kilograms)	200 POUNDS (91 kilograms)	240 POUNDS (109 kilograms)
Aerobics, low impact	365	455	545
Aerobics, water	292	364	436
Basketball game	584	728	872
Bicycling, < 10 mph, leisure	292	364	436
Bowling	219	273	327
Dancing, ballroom	219	273	327
Football, touch, flag, general	584	728	872
Golfing, carrying clubs	329	410	491
Hiking	438	546	654
Ice skating	511	637	763
Jogging, 5 mph	584	728	872
Racquetball, casual, general	511	637	763
Rope jumping	730	910	1,090
Rowing, stationary	511	637	763
Running, 8 mph	986	1,229	1,472
Skiing, cross-country	511	637	763
Skiing, downhill	365	455	545
Softball or baseball	365	455	545
Stair treadmill	657	819	981
Swimming, laps	511	637	763
Tennis, singles	584	728	872
Volleyball	292	364	436
Walking, 2 mph	183	228	273
Walking, 3.5 mph	277	346	414
Weightlifting	219	273	327

Based on Ainsworth BE, et al., *Medicine & Science in Sports & Exercise*, 2000

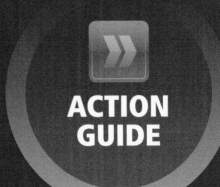

Action Guide to weight-loss barriers

Long-term success with a weight program sometimes follows a bumpy, uneven path. Many obstacles can keep you from achieving a more healthy weight.

Learning to identify potential roadblocks and confront personal temptations is an important part of being successful in losing weight. To make it past the rough spots, it's important to have strategies ready to guide your response as problems arise.

This easy-to-use action guide identifies common weight-loss barriers and practical strategies for overcoming them. If you find a strategy that helps you, include it with your weight-loss program.

The barriers are grouped into three categories: nutrition, physical activity and behaviors. To lose weight — and to maintain that weight loss — it's important that you address all of these components.

❱❱ Nutrition obstacle

I don't have time to make healthy meals.

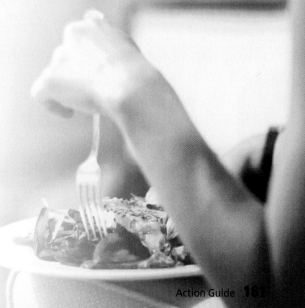 Having too little time to cook is a common obstacle for many people to eat healthy. At the same time, preparing your own meals is a key factor in weight control. Even when meal preparations are rushed, it's possible to find ways to eat healthier. Tasty, nutritious meals don't require a lot of cooking time, but they do require that you plan ahead.

❱❱ Strategies

Here are tips to help you eat well on a busy schedule.

+ Plan a week's worth of meals at a time. Make a detailed grocery list to eliminate last-minute trips to the grocery store.

+ Devote time on the weekend to preparing meals for the coming week. Consider making several meals and freezing them in meal-size batches.

+ Remember that healthy meals don't have to be complicated. Serve a fresh salad with fat-free dressing, a whole-grain roll and a piece of fruit.

+ Keep staple ingredients on hand for making basic meals. For example, you can quickly mix together rice, beans and spices for a Tex-Mex casserole.

+ Have family members help in the kitchen. Split up the tasks to save time.

+ On days when you don't have time to make a healthy meal, stop at a deli or grocery store and purchase a healthy sandwich, soup or prepared entree that's low in calories and low in fat.

)) Nutrition obstacle

I don't like to cook.

Not interested in becoming a gourmet chef? No problem. Many people are reluctant to change their diets because they worry that a healthier eating plan means spending too many hours in the kitchen or struggling with complicated recipes. Healthy eating doesn't require advanced cooking skills, and many healthy meals can be made with minimal time and effort.

)) Strategies

If you don't enjoy cooking, here are suggestions to help without a lot of culinary effort.

+ Purchase a cookbook that offers quick and easy healthy meals, or check one out at your local library.

+ Base your meals on fresh fruits and vegetables, none of which takes much preparation or cooking time.

+ Try out a variety of cooking techniques. You might not like baking, but microwaving or grilling may be your thing.

+ Be creative. Use shortcuts such as prepackaged salad greens or raw vegetables, or precooked lean meats.

+ Eat out or order in. It's OK to eat at a restaurant, order in dinner or buy something ready to eat on your way home as long as you choose items that are healthy and you eat moderate portions.

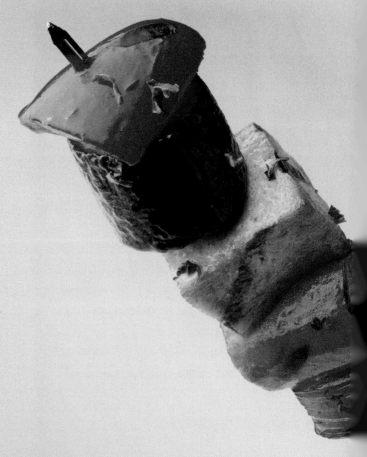

)) Nutrition obstacle

I don't like vegetables and fruits.

Some people find vegetables and fruits boring. Common opinions hold that vegetables and fruits don't have much flavor or that they all taste the same. Not true! Vegetables and fruits are tasty — you just have to know which kinds you prefer and how to prepare them. Much of what you eat is conditioned — over time, you've learned to like it. You still can learn to enjoy new foods, such as vegetables and fruits.

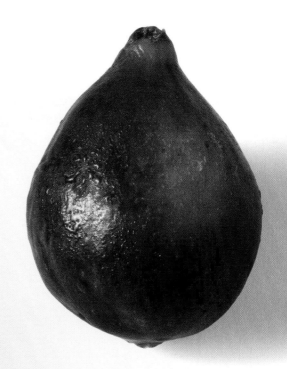

)) Strategies

You can experiment with vegetables and fruits. Here are some suggestions.

+ Keep in mind that you don't need to like all varieties of vegetables and fruits, just some of them.

+ Instead of the familiar apples, grapes and oranges, buy fresh fruits that you haven't tried before. How about kiwis, mangoes, papayas, Bing cherries and apricots?

+ Try using more vegetables and fruits in other foods and recipes: Add vegetables to one of your favorite soups, replace some of the hamburger in casseroles with vegetables, add peppers and onions to your pizza, include fresh fruit with your morning cereal, mix fruit with yogurt or cottage cheese.

+ Try different ways of preparation. For example, grill pineapple or fruit kebabs. Make fruit smoothies with blueberries and low-fat yogurt.

+ If you don't care for raw vegetables, lightly cook them and see if you prefer the softer texture. Sprinkle them with herbs for flavor.

)) Nutrition obstacle

Healthy foods, such as fresh produce and fish, are expensive. I can't afford them.

Although fresh produce and fish can be expensive, your overall grocery bill may actually be less because you're eating less of other foods, such as chips, cookies and ice cream. These processed foods can also be costly. Plus, you may find that you're eating more meals at home and fewer in restaurants — this, too, can save money.

)) Strategies

Here are suggestions to prevent the calories in food you buy from adding up at the grocery store.

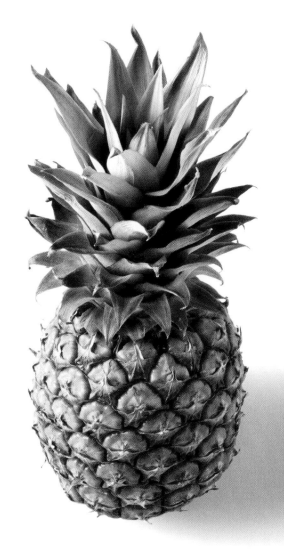

+ A report indicates that, with smart planning, it's possible to obtain your recommended daily servings of fruits and vegetables at a very limited price. Check your options at the grocery store and watch for specials.

+ Buy grains such as oatmeal and brown rice in bulk. Food co-ops are often good at offering foods in bulk.

+ Visit farmers markets for summertime deals. You can usually pick up the freshest produce at the lowest prices.

+ Consider growing some of your own produce. It's not as hard as you think. If you don't have room for a garden, you can grow items such as tomatoes and peppers in outdoor pots.

+ Eat simple meals sometimes. A peanut butter sandwich made with whole wheat bread or a bowl of soup and a few pieces of fruit don't cost much.

)) Nutrition obstacle

My family doesn't like to try new foods, and it's too much work to make two different meals.

Family support is important when you're trying to lose weight, but don't let your family stop you from trying something new or exploring different ways of preparing favorite foods. When your family sees you enjoying a meal, your good habits may eventually rub off on them, too. People underestimate their ability to change their tastes. For example, when people first try skim or low-fat milk, they often say that it tastes like water. But after they stick with it for a while, most of these same people say that whole milk tastes too rich.

)) Strategies

Here are changes that may help both you and your family to enjoy tastes in common and get on the same healthy track.

+ Take it slow. Don't try to overhaul your family's diet overnight. Make a few small changes at a time. Eventually, these small changes add up, and soon you'll all be following a healthier eating plan.

+ Offer a favorite dish that's prepared using a different cooking method. For example, instead of frying pork chops or chicken breasts, bake or grill them.

+ Involve your family in meal planning. Ask family members what they'd like to try that's different and healthy. If they can choose, they might be more willing to experiment.

+ Keep more fruits and vegetables in the house, and keep fruit in a location where it's visible. When looking for a snack, make it easy to grab bananas, pears or grapes.

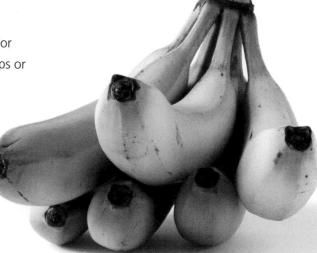

▶▶ Nutrition obstacle

I can't resist certain foods, such as chocolate and candy.

To achieve a goal, you have to be flexible. As you prepare a healthy-eating plan, ask yourself how to fit occasional sweets or junk food into the plan without destroying your overall weight goal. Instead of avoiding these kinds of foods, give yourself permission to eat them on occasion and in moderation. If you try to avoid these foods completely, you'll feel deprived when you can't have them, which leads to disillusionment and to binge eating.

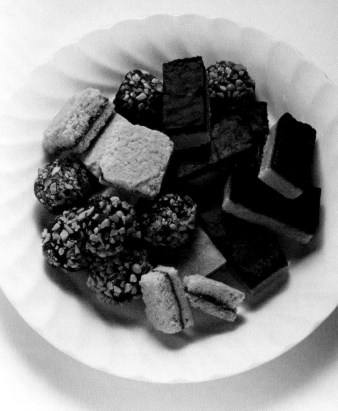

▶▶ Strategies

Here are suggestions that may help you incorporate favorite unhealthy foods into your healthy eating plan.

+ Plan ahead for the events occurring during the week that put you around sweets and junk food. In appropriate situations — such as going out to dinner with friends — enjoy some of your favorite foods in moderate portions.

+ Know that once you've sampled a favorite food, you may crave more. So it's important to determine in advance how much you'll eat and stick to that portion.

+ Eat healthy foods beforehand so that when it comes time to enjoy a favorite sweet or junk food, you won't be as hungry and will eat less.

+ Don't keep chocolate or junk food at home. If you get an urge to eat such foods, but you have to go out and buy them first, the urge might pass. If you do buy chocolate or junk food, buy it in small amounts, such as single servings.

)) Nutrition obstacle

I travel a lot, and I often have to eat at airports, hotels or events.

It can be more difficult to eat healthy when traveling, but it's certainly not impossible. You can find healthy choices when you're away from home. Part of the solution may be your mindset. Avoid rationalizations such as, "I'm traveling, so I'll have to eat whatever is available."

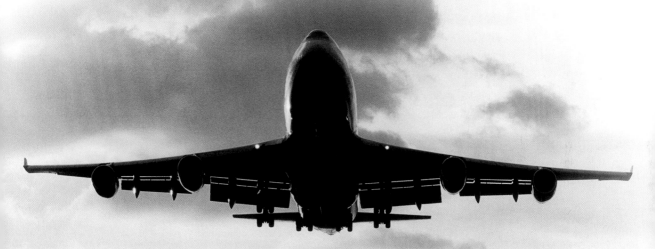

)) Strategies

Eating well on the road often requires a little planning before you travel.

+ If you travel by car, pack a cooler with healthy foods, such as sandwiches, yogurt, fruit and raw vegetables.

+ If you travel by plane, pack snacks such as nuts and fruit in your carry-on bag.

+ Ask employees at hotels or conferences about local restaurants that have healthy foods on their menus, or that offer grilled or broiled foods in addition to fried foods. You might also ask if there's a grocery store nearby where you can purchase fruit and easy-to-fix items.

+ At business events, use portion control. Allow yourself small servings of some higher calorie foods so that you don't feel deprived, but eat larger servings of lower calorie foods.

+ Focus your mind on how eating healthy will give you the strength and energy you'll need for your trip.

)) Nutrition obstacle

Since I'm not hungry in the morning, I often skip breakfast.

Breakfast is an important meal. Research suggests that people who eat breakfast reach their dietary goals and manage their weight better than do people who don't eat breakfast. Even if you're not hungry, try to eat a little something in the morning. Just as your body became accustomed to not eating breakfast, it can get used to eating it again. A good breakfast also helps keep you from becoming ravenously hungry later in the day, so you won't eat as much.

)) Strategies

To eat a good breakfast, even if you're not hungry, try these tips.

+ Change gradually. Have breakfast on two mornings at first, and three mornings a little later. Your eventual goal is to eat breakfast every day.

+ If time is an issue, do some preparation the evening before. Place a box of cereal, a bowl and a spoon on the table. Or have a breakfast shake ready that comes in a can or that you mix yourself.

+ Keep on hand food that you can carry with you to eat in the car, on the train or bus, or at work. Convenient on-the-go foods include apples, bananas, whole-grain bagels and low-fat yogurt in single-serving containers.

+ If you don't like traditional breakfast foods, fix a breakfast sandwich.

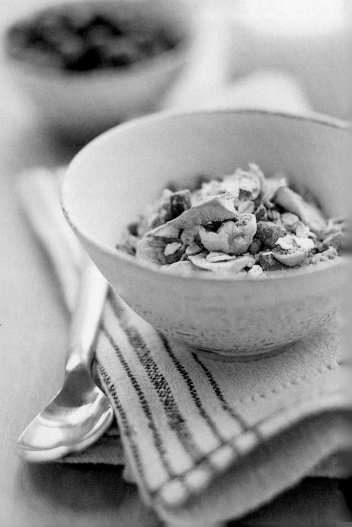

)) Nutrition obstacle

I'm not good at menu planning. I never have the right ingredients around the house to make a healthy meal.

It always helps if you plan ahead, but you can wing it and still eat well. Remember that healthy eating doesn't have to be complicated or involve hard-to-find ingredients. When you go to the grocery store, stock up on some of the basics. If you have on hand foods and ingredients such as the ones suggested below, you'll be able to prepare a good meal.

)) Strategies

Here are examples of good foods and ingredients to always have on hand.

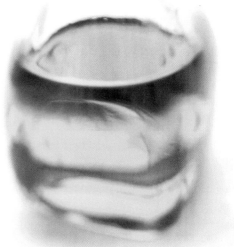

+ Plenty of fruits and vegetables, including canned tomato products and vegetable soups and broth.

+ Lentils and beans such as black beans, kidney beans and garbanzos.

+ Low-fat or fat-free milk, low-fat or fat-free cottage cheese, and reduced-fat cheeses.

+ Kitchen staples that you know you'll frequently use, such as salt and pepper. Add to your weekly shopping lists fresh produce, meat, dairy and bakery goods.

+ Skinless chicken and turkey, unbreaded fish, extra-lean ground beef, and round or sirloin beef cuts.

+ Cooking spray, olive oil and trans fat-free margarine.

+ Condiments, seasonings and spreads such as low-fat or fat-free salad dressings, herbs, spices, flavored vinegars, hummus and salsa.

+ Whole-grain bread, bagels and pita bread, low-fat tortillas, oatmeal, brown and white rice, whole-grain pasta, and whole-grain cereals that aren't pre-sweetened.

)) Physical activity obstacle

I don't have time to exercise.

Much as with mealtimes, time for exercise is a common obstacle. With creativity and planning, you can overcome this obstacle. Perhaps you have more time than you realize. For example, the average American watches four hours of television each day. Add to that the time you may spend surfing the Web or going on minor errands in the car, and there's bound to be extra time for physical activity. In most cases, time really isn't the issue, rather it's a matter of priorities. To become more physically active, it may be that you need to give up another habit.

)) Strategies

If you can't find at least 30 minutes during your day to exercise, look for 10-minute windows. Exercising for 10 minutes three times a day is beneficial, too. Here are strategies you might try.

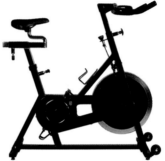

+ Walk for 10 minutes over your lunch hour, or get up a few minutes earlier in the morning and go for a short walk.

+ Take the stairs instead of the elevator, at least for a few floors.

+ Take regular activity breaks. Get up from your desk to stretch and walk around.

+ Instead of always looking for the short-cut from one destination to another, look for opportunities to walk and get more physical activity in your day.

+ Develop a routine that you can do at home. While watching your favorite television program or reading, walk on a treadmill, ride a stationary bicycle or use an elliptical machine.

+ Use the community pool to swim laps or do water workouts.

+ Schedule time with a friend to do physical activities together on a regular basis.

+ While your child is at soccer practice or taking piano lessons, go for a walk or jog.

» Physical activity obstacle

I'm too tired to exercise.

Maybe that's because you're not exercising enough. Many people find they're less tired once they're involved with a regular exercise program. That's because regular physical activity gives you more energy and because fatigue is more often mental than it is physical. If you're fatigued due to stress, exercise is a great stress reliever.

» Strategies

To incorporate more physical activity into your day, try these tips.

+ Begin with just five to 10 minutes of activity. Keep in mind that a little activity is better than none. And once you start, chances are you'll keep going for the full 10 minutes — if not longer.

+ Exercise in the morning. This will give you more energy throughout the day.

+ When you get home from work, don't sit down to watch television or use the computer. Instead, put on your walking shoes as soon as you arrive home and go for a walk.

+ Keep motivational messages where you need them to remind you of your goal.

)) Physical activity obstacle

I don't like to exercise.

People who don't like to exercise generally view physical activity as painful or boring. It doesn't have to be either. From among the many forms of physical activity, you're bound to find something enjoyable. You need to experiment. Find something that piques your interest and try it out.

)) Strategies

Here are things you can do to help make exercise more enjoyable.

+ Try not to focus on exercise only. Think of enjoyable things to do in which you're physically active, such as working in your flower garden or helping a friend with a building project. How you frame physical activity in your mind can make a big difference.

+ Take advantage of introductory classes or exercise videos to learn basic skills and techniques.

+ Mix things up. Don't feel tied to one activity, such as walking. On occasion, try biking or swimming instead. For more ideas on different activities, see pages 96-97 and 172-179.

+ Listen to music while you exercise. Upbeat music can rev you up and make your workout seem easier. It can also make the time pass more quickly.

+ Focus on the benefits of activity instead of the activity itself. Think of your workout time as personal time for you. Reflect on your goals and remind yourself how good it'll feel to achieve them.

+ Exercise with a friend or in a group. That way, you can socialize while you exercise, which may make the time go faster and the task seem less boring or painful.

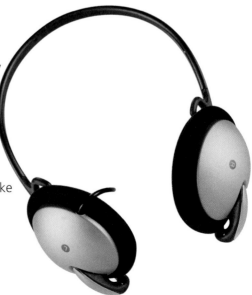

)) Physical activity obstacle

I'm too old to exercise. I might hurt myself.

You're never too old or out of shape to be physically active, and it's never too late to start. Moderate physical activity can help you achieve or maintain a healthy weight. Moderate physical activity can also help delay age-associated illnesses and conditions such as heart disease, high blood pressure, diabetes and bone loss.

)) Strategies

If you haven't been active, it's important to see your doctor before starting exercise, especially if you have some health concerns. Once your doctor gives the OK, here are suggestions for getting started.

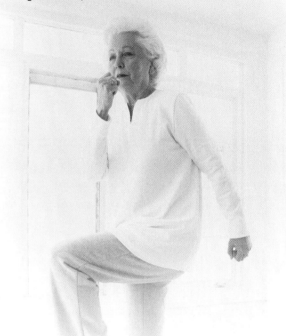

+ Start slowly and give your body a chance to get used to increased activity. Once you're accustomed to the change, gradually increase your activity level.

+ Walking is a good starter exercise. Other options include a stationary bike with no resistance or water exercise.

+ Consider light-resistance exercises, such as the use of elastic bands, for strength training. Studies indicate that even people in their 80s can double their strength at this level of exercise.

+ Do things you enjoy. Activities such as dancing and gardening can provide effective workouts.

+ Stretch. Staying flexible is key to improving or maintaining a full range of motion in your joints and muscles. It's best to do stretching exercises after a brief warm-up period of light activity.

+ Muscle soreness after exercise is common, especially if it's a new activity. Pain during exercise sends a different signal and may require you to stop. For more on exercise red flags, see page 175.

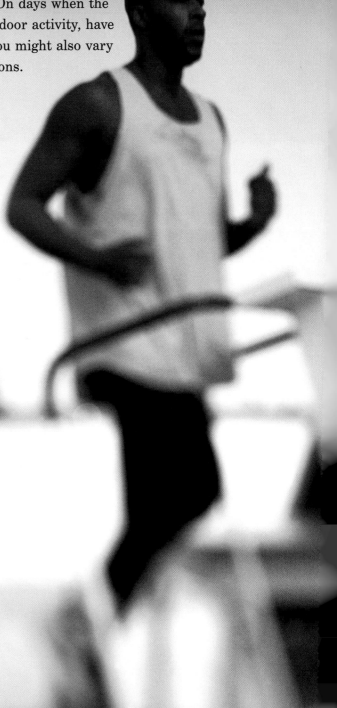

)) Physical activity obstacle

I don't like to exercise when it's cold, rainy or hot.

Choose activities that you can do regardless of the weather, and be flexible with your exercise routine. On days when the weather isn't conducive to your normal outdoor activity, have plans ready for alternate indoor activity. You might also vary your exercise routine according to the seasons.

)) Strategies

Here are some suggestions to consider.

+ Have options for moving your routine indoors. If you bicycle, cycle inside on a stationary bicycle. If you like to walk, walk indoors at a nearby mall or school.

+ Be willing to try something different. Instead of jogging, do indoor aerobics or strength exercises.

+ Swimming in the summer provides a great aerobic workout while also keeping you cool.

+ In colder climates, take advantage of activities such as ice-skating, snowshoeing or cross-country skiing.

+ Check out the local health club. Some don't require that you have a membership but rather allow you to pay per visit.

)) Physical activity obstacle

I worry that other people will think I look funny when I exercise.

Try putting aside such thoughts. Most active people will give you credit for exercising and not make fun of you. Ask yourself which is more important: avoiding feeling possible embarrassment or losing weight. Once you get started, you may find that exercising isn't as embarrassing as you thought it would be.

)) Strategies

If you're concerned about exercising in front of others, consider these suggestions.

+ Most of your self-consciousness will disappear as exercise becomes more routine and you become more confident.

+ Sign up for an exercise class that includes other people trying to lose weight.

+ Buy an exercise video or an exercise machine, such as a stationary bicycle or treadmill, so that you can work out in the privacy of your own home.

+ Exercise early in the morning or late in the evening, when fewer people are around.

+ Ask an exercise professional to demonstrate proper technique and provide information on appropriate exercises so that you can feel confident in your abilities.

)) Physical activity obstacle
I travel a lot, so exercise is inconvenient.

Travel, whether for business or pleasure, doesn't have to interrupt your exercise routine. It's easier than you may think to incorporate physical activity into your trips away from home. Doing so can bolster your energy level and help you better handle the stress of travel.

)) Strategies
Healthy habits travel easily. Here are strategies for staying fit on the road.

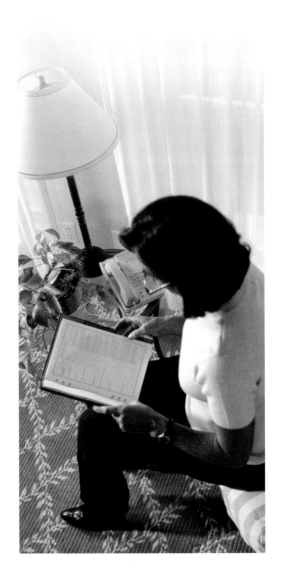

+ Contact your hotel and ask about fitness facilities on-site or nearby. Knowing what's available will help you pack the right workout clothes.

+ Remember that walking can be done almost anywhere. Walk around the airport terminal while you're waiting to board a flight. When you're driving, make an occasional stop to get out and walk around a rest area.

+ Do exercises in your hotel room. Pack an exercise band or jump-rope or do exercises that don't require equipment, such as sit-ups or squats.

+ If you're able to, rent a bicycle in your new location and go sightseeing. Or, check with your hotel on neighborhoods to explore on foot.

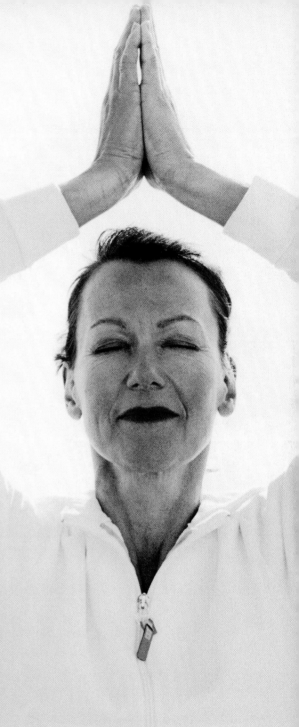

)) Physical activity obstacle

I can't exercise because of painful arthritis in my joints.

For many people with chronic pain, exercise can be very beneficial. Physical activity can help you manage the symptoms of other chronic conditions. In the case of arthritis, proper exercise can help you better maintain joint mobility.

)) Strategies

The key is knowing which exercises are helpful to your condition and which are harmful. If you have arthritis:

+ Try water exercises. The buoyancy of water takes the weight off your joints. You can swim laps on your own or you might try a water aerobics class.

+ Use a stationary or recumbent bicycle, which takes pressure off your knees.

+ Consider joining a basic yoga or tai chi class to increase strength and flexibility in your joints.

+ See a physical therapist who can offer recommendations on the best type of exercises for you and teach you how to do them properly to avoid injury and further pain.

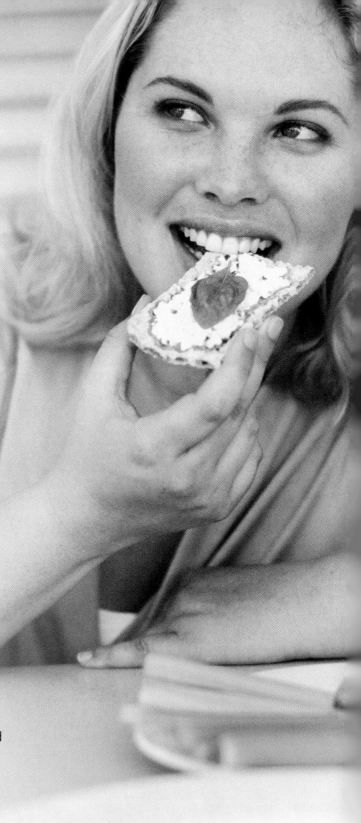

)) Physical activity obstacle

Exercise makes me hungry.

You may find that about an hour or
so after you've finished working out,
you're hungry. Studies also show
that people tend to eat a little more
after they start exercising regularly.
However, you're typically burning
more calories from the new exercise than you're taking in with the
increased eating. There's certainly
nothing wrong with eating after exercise, but you don't want to negate all
of the potential benefits by loading up
mindlessly on high-calorie snacks.

)) Strategies

Here are suggestions for maintaining the
benefits of physical activity, while also
satisfying your hunger following exercise.

+ Before you exercise, eat foods that stick
  with you longer, such as whole-grain
  bread, cereal, pasta and brown rice.

+ Before you exercise, prepare a light,
  healthy snack for after your workout,
  such as fruit, yogurt or whole-grain
  crackers.

+ Drink plenty of water before, during and
  after your workout.

›› Behaviors obstacle

I have trouble controlling how much I eat.

For many people, a major struggle in reaching a healthy weight is learning how to eat less. Part of the problem is that they don't have a realistic idea of what constitutes a serving. In an era of jumbo meals, supersizing and free refills, overgenerous portions of food and beverages have become the norm. In addition, eating habits that you learned from a young age — that it's OK to have seconds, that you should clean your plate, that dessert must always follow a meal — can be difficult to break. But difficult doesn't mean impossible.

›› Strategies

You can train your body to feel full with less food, in the same way that your body became accustomed to needing more food to feel full. Try these suggestions.

+ Serve meals already dished onto plates instead of placing serving bowls on the table. This requires you to think twice before having a second portion.

+ Try using a smaller plate or bowl to make less food seem like more.

+ Eat slowly. When you eat too fast, your brain doesn't get the signal that you're full until after you've overeaten.

+ Eat the foods that are healthy and low in calories first, before turning your attention to higher calorie foods.

+ Focus on your meal and on your company. Watching television, reading or working while you eat too often leads to mindless eating.

+ Stop eating as soon as you begin to feel full. You don't need to clean your plate.

+ Designate one area of the house to eat meals and only sit there when you eat.

+ If you're still hungry after finishing what's on your plate, nibble on something that's low in calories, such as fresh vegetables, fruit or crackers.

+ Portion sizes in restaurants can be two to three times the amount you need. Request a carry-out container to take the excess home for another meal.

)) Behaviors obstacle

I've tried to lose weight before, but it didn't work. Now, I don't have confidence that it'll work this time.

For many people, losing weight will be one of life's most difficult challenges. Don't be discouraged if you've tried losing weight in the past and you weren't able to — or you lost weight but gained it all back. Many people experiment with several different weight-loss plans before they find an approach that works.

)) Strategies

Following these tips may help you succeed this time around.

+ Think of losing weight as a positive experience, not a negative one. Approaching weight loss with a positive attitude will help you succeed.

+ Set realistic expectations for yourself. Focus on behavioral changes and don't focus too much on weight changes.

+ Use problem-solving techniques. Write down the obstacles that you experienced in previous attempts to lose weight, and come up with strategies for dealing with those obstacles.

+ Make small, not drastic, changes to your lifestyle. Adjustments that are too intense or vigorous can make you uncomfortable and cause you to give up.

+ Accept the fact that you'll have setbacks. Believe in yourself. Instead of giving up entirely, simply start fresh the next day.

>> Behaviors obstacle

I eat when I'm stressed, depressed or bored.

Sometimes your most intense longings for food happen right when you're at your weakest emotional points. Many people turn to food for comfort — be it consciously or unconsciously — when they're dealing with difficult problems or looking for something to distract their minds.

>> Strategies

To help keep food out of your mood, try these suggestions.

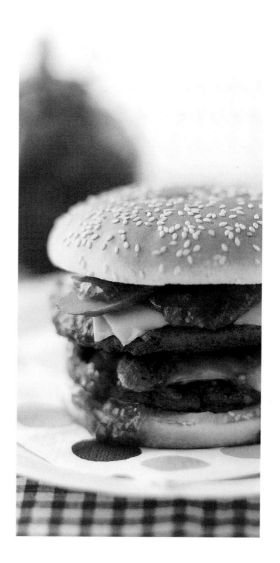

+ Try to distract yourself from eating by calling a friend, running an errand or going for a walk. When you can focus your mind on something else, the food cravings quickly go away.

+ Don't keep comfort foods in the house. If you turn to high-fat, high-calorie foods whenever you're upset or depressed, make an effort to get rid of them.

+ Identify your mood. Often the urge to eat can be attributed to a specific mood and not to physical hunger.

+ When you feel down, make an attempt to replace negative thoughts with positive ones. For example, write down all of the positive qualities about yourself and what you plan to achieve by losing weight.

)) Behaviors obstacle

I have a hard time not eating when I'm watching television, a movie or a live sporting event.

There's nothing inherently wrong with eating while watching a show, film or live event, but when you're distracted, you tend to eat mindlessly — which typically translates into eating more than you intended to eat. If you're unable to break this habit, at least make sure you're munching on something low in calories.

)) Strategies

Here are suggestions you might consider.

+ If you're at a theater or stadium, order a small bag of popcorn with no butter and work on it slowly.

+ Eat something healthy before you leave home so that you're not extremely hungry when you arrive.

+ Drink water or a calorie-free beverage instead of having a snack.

+ Try to reduce the amount of time that you spend watching television each day. Studies show that TV watching contributes to increased weight.

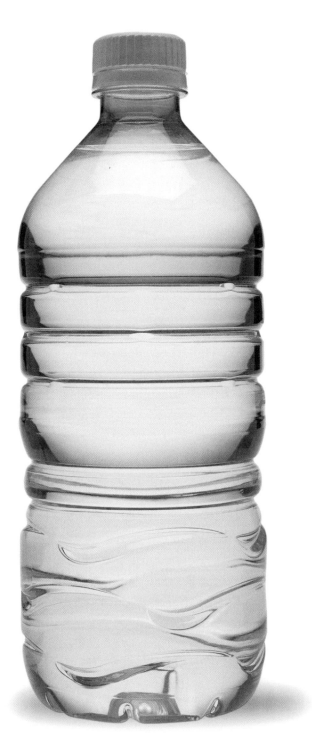

)) Behaviors obstacle

When I go to parties, I can't resist all of the snacks and hors d'oeuvres.

In most social situations where food is involved, the key is to treat yourself to a few of your favorite hors d'oeuvres, in moderation. If you try to resist the food, your craving will only get stronger and harder to control. By following a few simple strategies, you can enjoy yourself without overeating.

)) Strategies

Next time you step up to the hors d'oeuvre table, try these strategies.

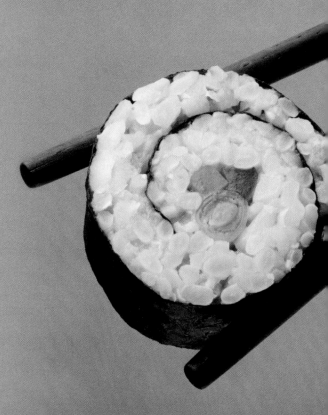

+ Make only one trip and be selective. Decide ahead of time how much you'll eat and choose foods you really want.

+ Treat yourself to one or two samples of high-calorie or fatty foods. Fill up on vegetables and fruits, if you can.

+ Take only small portions. A taste may be all that you need to satisfy your craving.

+ Nibble. If you eat slowly, you'll likely eat less — but don't nibble all night long.

+ Don't stand next to or sit near the hors d'oeuvre table. As the old saying goes, "Out of sight, out of mind."

+ Eat something healthy before you arrive. If you arrive hungry, you'll be more inclined to overeat.

❱❱ Behaviors obstacle

I'm a late-night snacker.

Avoid eating late at night because loading up on calories right before bed only intensifies the challenge of not overeating. There's less chance for you to be active and burn off those calories until next morning. It's better to eat during the day so that your body has plenty of time to digest the food before you go to bed.

❱❱ Strategies

Here are suggestions if you often find yourself battling the late-night munchies.

+ Make sure you eat three good meals during the day, including a good break-fast. This will help reduce the urge to snack late at night, simply because you won't be so hungry.

+ Don't keep snack foods around the house that may tempt you. If you get late-night munchies, eat fruits, vegeta-bles or other healthy snacks.

+ Find something else to keep you busy in the hours before bedtime, such as listening to music or exercising. Your snacking may be more of a mindless habit than actual hunger.

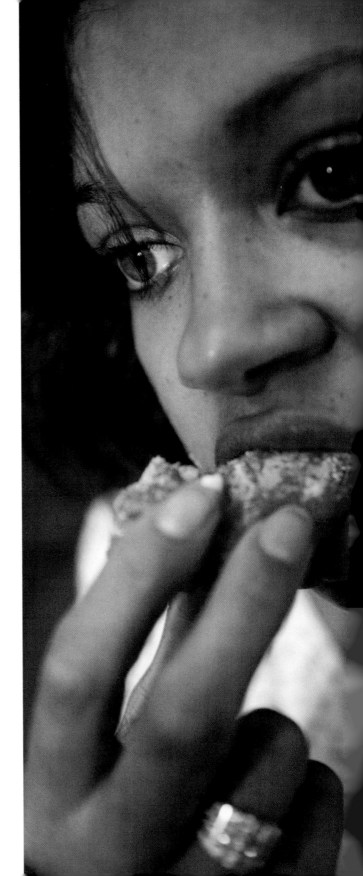

)) Behaviors obstacle

When I lapse from my eating plan, it's hard for me to get back on track.

Lapses happen. Many times a minor slip — a busy day when you couldn't find the time to eat right or get exercise — leads to more slips. That doesn't mean, though, that you've failed and all is lost. Instead of beating yourself up over a lapse, accept that you're going to experience bumps along the way and put the incident behind you. Everyone has lapses. Think back to the initial steps you took when you first began your weight program and put them to use again to help you get back on track.

)) Strategies

Here are suggestions to prevent a lapse from turning into a full-blown collapse.

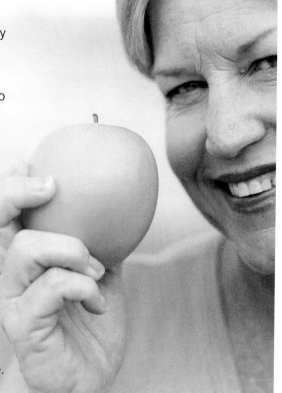

+ Convince yourself that lapses happen and that every day is a fresh opportunity to start over again.

+ Guilt from the initial lapse often leads to more lapses. Being prepared for them and having a plan to deal with them is important to your success.

+ Keep your response simple. Focus on the things that you know you can do and stick with them. Gradually add more healthy changes until you're back on track.

+ Open up an old food record and follow it. Use those meals like a menu to help get you back to a healthy eating routine.

)) Behaviors obstacle

I get frustrated when I lose just a pound or two after I've tried really hard all week.

Many people long for a secret potion or magic pill that will quickly remove excess weight. Unfortunately, such a remedy doesn't exist. Losing 1 or 2 pounds a week may be frustrating if your expectations are high. But slow and steady is a healthy way to go, and by doing it this way, the weight is much more likely to stay off.

)) Strategies

Follow these tips to keep yourself on track.

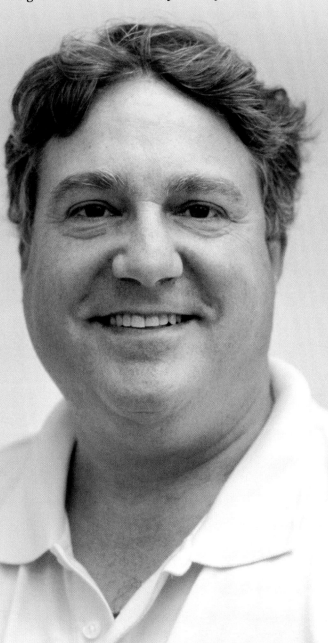

+ Don't focus all of your attention on the bathroom scale. Concentrate on eating better and exercising more.

+ Don't consider yourself to be "on a diet." Try to adopt a positive outlook with the goal of a healthier lifestyle.

+ Make a list of all the benefits of losing weight, such as having more energy, improving your health and feeling better about yourself. Refer to this list if your motivation wanes.

+ Don't use life's ups and downs as an excuse to quit. If stressful events occur, cut yourself some slack if you need to, but stay with the program.

+ Remind yourself that losing 1 to 2 pounds a week equates to about 50 to 100 pounds a year!

❱❱ Behaviors obstacle

I don't like my body image.

How you feel about your body can be central to how you feel about yourself. Many people despair when comparing the way they look to the way they feel they should look. This results in emotional hurt. Having a positive view of your body — no matter how imperfect it may be — is critical to success. To feel good about what you're achieving by losing weight and improving your health, you have to feel good about your body.

❱❱ Strategies

Here are suggestions to help you view your body in a more positive light.

+ Think of your body as a gift. It allows you to live, move, achieve and experience pleasure. If you focus on the good things about your body, it becomes more of a friend and less of an adversary.

+ Don't equate body image with self-esteem. The assumption that how you look is who you are can sabotage your weight goals. Your appearance is only one aspect of your life. You can be a success at many things, regardless of appearance (or how you think you appear). Focus on the things that you're good at.

+ Don't avoid looking at your body. Many people avoid mirrors and windows so that they won't have to look at their reflections. Instead, consider your reflection as a way to measure success.

+ Write a list of positive things about yourself and add to it often. Refer to the list when you need support. In addition, post self-affirming messages ("I'm strong and resilient!") on your bathroom mirror, in your car or at your desk at work.

+ Spend time with people who are positive and supportive of your efforts to lose weight and live healthy.

+ Remember that appearance can be independent of health. Some people are slender but deal with increased health risks. Conversely, other people may not have a picture-perfect appearance, but their attitudes and spirits are wonderful. Beauty comes from within. When you feel good about yourself, your positive outlook will shine through.

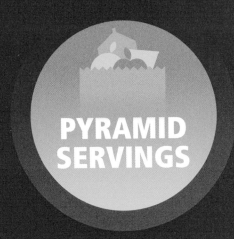

PYRAMID
SERVINGS

Pyramid servings at a glance

In Chapter 6 you determined your daily goals for servings
from each of the Mayo Clinic Healthy Weight Pyramid food
groups. To achieve those goals, you need to know how much
food is in a serving. The lists in this section can help.

Visual guide to servings sizes
See larger chart on page 73.

1 Vegetable serving =
1 baseball

1 Fruit serving =
1 tennis ball

OK, you've realized that not all the foods you eat fit the visual cues from "Quick guide to serving sizes" on page 73. How can you determine pyramid servings? Here's a place to start.

The first part of this section is subdivided according to food groups. It lists individual foods in amounts that equal a single serving. So, by checking the lists, you'll know that if you eat a medium tomato or a half-cup of pasta, it's going to be one serving.

The second part involves "mixed foods," which generally include more than one ingredient (and more than one food group). The separate entries break down servings from the different food groups. So, by checking the lists, you'll know that a peanut butter and jelly sandwich includes carbohydrate, fat and sweet servings.

Important: The serving sizes shown in these lists are "ready to eat" — cooked or raw.

Figuring out your servings

You've just made a small salad topped with olive oil and seasoning. Figuring out your servings begins with your best estimate of the amounts. A good guess is generally good enough.

1 You guess from the size of your bowl that it's filled with about 1 cup of lettuce. In the vegetable listing, you see that 2 cups of lettuce is one serving, so:
+ **1 cup of lettuce in your bowl = ½ vegetable serving**

2 You note that you used about one-half of a carrot, cucumber and tomato in the salad. The list indicates that any of these medium-size vegetables is one serving, so:
+ **½ each of the carrot, cucumber and tomato = 1½ vegetable servings**

3 You learn from the fats listing that 1 teaspoon of olive oil is one serving, which is about what you used. The small amount of seasoning isn't enough to count.

So, the servings breakdown for your salad is:
+ 2 vegetable servings
+ 1 fat serving

---

1 Carbohydrate serving =
1 hockey puck

1 Protein/Dairy serving =
1 deck of cards or less

1 Fat serving =
1 to 2 dice

Vegetables

Item (25 calories per serving)	One serving is
★ Alfalfa sprouts	1 cup
★ Artichoke bud	½ bud
★ Artichoke hearts	½ cup
★ Arugula	2 cups
★ Asparagus, cooked	½ cup or 6 spears
★ Bamboo shoots	½ cup
★ Bean sprouts	1 cup
Beans, green, canned or frozen	⅔ cup
★ Beans, green, fresh	⅔ cup
★ Beets	½ cup sliced
★ Bell pepper, green, red or yellow	1 cup sliced or 1 medium
★ Broccoli	1 cup florets
★ Brussels sprouts	½ cup or 4 sprouts
★ Cabbage, bok choy, Chinese	2 cups chopped or 1 cup cooked
★ Cabbage, green or red	1 cup chopped or ½ cup cooked
★ Carrots	½ cup baby or 1 medium
★ Cauliflower	1 cup florets (about 8)
★ Celery	1 cup diced or 4 medium stalks
★ Collard greens, cooked	½ cup
★ Cucumber	1 cup sliced or 1 medium
★ Eggplant, cooked	1 cup cubed
★ Jicama (yambean)	½ cup sliced
★ Kale, cooked	⅔ cup

★ **Blue star indicates the best choices.**

Vegetables are nutritional powerhouses, but they're too often treated as accompaniments or side dishes to the main course. Use their vibrant flavors, colors and textures to expand their role in your diet.

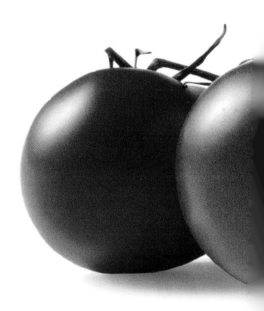

Vegetables

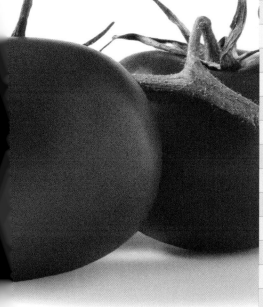

FROM THE DIETITIAN

Looking for corn and potatoes? Many people may consider them vegetables but, due to their nutritional makeup, you'll find them listed with carbohydrates. Green peas are listed with protein and dairy items.

Item (25 calories per serving)	One serving is
★ Leek, cooked	½ cup
★ Lettuce, iceberg	2 cups shredded
★ Lettuce, romaine	2 cups chopped
Marinara and pizza sauce, canned	2 tablespoons
★ Mushrooms	1 cup whole (about 6 medium)
Mushrooms, canned	½ cup
★ Okra	½ cup or 3 pods
★ Onions, sweet, white or red	½ cup sliced
★ Onions, young green (scallions)	¾ cup or 8 shoots
★ Radishes	25 medium
Salsa, vegetable	¼ cup
★ Shallots	3 tablespoons chopped
★ Spinach	2 cups
★ Spinach, cooked	½ cup
★ Squash, summer	¾ cup sliced
★ Tomatillo	½ cup diced or 2 medium
★ Tomato	1 medium
★ Tomato, cherry or grape	1 cup (about 8)
Tomato, stewed, canned	½ cup
Tomato paste, canned	2 tablespoons
Tomato sauce, canned	⅓ cup
Water chestnuts, sliced, canned	¾ cup
★ Zucchini, fresh or cooked	¾ cup

★ **Blue star indicates the best choices.**

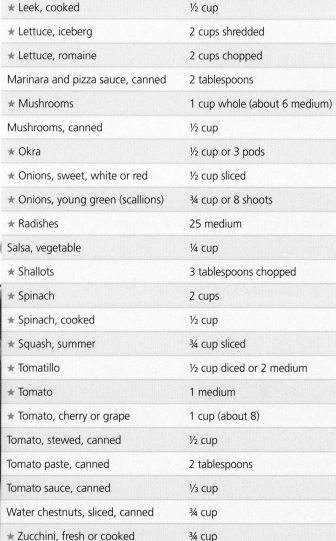

Fruits

Item (60 calories per serving)	One serving is
★ Apple	1 small
Apple, dried	⅓ cup
Applesauce, sweetened	⅓ cup
★ Applesauce, unsweetened	½ cup
★ Apricot	4 whole or 8 dried halves
★ Banana	1 small
★ Berries, mixed	¾ cup
★ Blackberries	1 cup
★ Blueberries	¾ cup
★ Breadfruit	¼ cup
★ Cantaloupe (muskmelon)	1 cup cubed or ⅓ small melon
★ Cherries	15 fruits
★ Clementine	2 small
Dates	3 fruits
★ Figs	2 small
Figs, dried	3 small
★ Grapefruit	¾ cup sections or ½ large
★ Grapes, seedless, red or green	1 cup (about 30)
★ Guava	2 fruits or ½ cup
★ Honeydew melon	1 cup cubed
★ Kiwi	1 large
★ Lemon	3 medium
★ Litchi (lychee)	10 fruits or ½ cup
Mandarin orange, canned in juice	¾ cup sections

★   **Blue star indicates the best choices.**

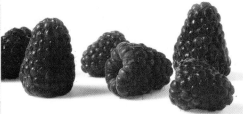

🍴 FROM THE DIETITIAN

The principle of unlimited fruit servings in The Mayo Clinic Diet does not apply to dried varieties such as apples, raisins and dates. That's because when the fruits dry, they shrink — so just a little piece of dried fruit contains a lot of calories! Dried fruit is still healthy but follow the recommended serving sizes listed in these pages

Fruits

Certain foods, such as cranberries and rhubarb, are tart and usually prepared with lots of added sugar before eating. You'll find the serving sizes for these foods listed with sweets. You'll find many juices in the beverage list.

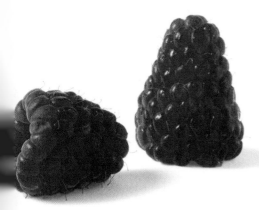

Item (60 calories per serving)	One serving is
★ Mango	½ cup diced
★ Melon balls	1 cup (about 8 balls)
Mixed fruit, dried	3 tablespoons
Mixed fruit cocktail, canned	¾ cup
★ Nectarine	1 fruit
★ Orange	¾ cup sections or 1 medium
★ Papaya	1 cup cubes or ½ medium
★ Peach	¾ cup sections or 1 medium
Peach, canned in juice	½ cup slices
★ Pear	1 small
Pear, canned in juice	½ cup halves
★ Pineapple	½ cup cubed or 2 rings
Pineapple, canned in juice	⅓ cup crushed or 2 rings
★ Plums	2 fruits
★ Pomegranate	½ cup
Prunes	3 fruits
★ Quince	1 fruit (about 3 ounces)
Raisins	2 tablespoons
★ Raspberries	1 cup
★ Star fruit or carambola	2 medium to large
★ Strawberries	1½ cups whole
★ Tangerine	1 large or 2 small
★ Watermelon	1¼ cups cubed or small wedge

★   **Blue star indicates the best choices.**

Carbohydrates

Item (70 calories per serving)	One serving is
Animal crackers	6 crackers
Bagel, cinnamon-raisin	½ bagel (3-inch)
★ Bagel, whole-grain	½ bagel (3-inch)
★ Barley, cooked	⅓ cup
Biscuits, plain or buttermilk, from dry mix	1 small
Bread, white or sourdough	1 slice
★ Bread, whole-grain	1 slice
★ Bread, whole-wheat white	1 slice
Breadsticks, crispy	2 sticks (6 to 8 inches)
★ Bulgur, cooked	½ cup
★ Bun or roll, whole-grain	1 small
★ Cereal, cold, bran-type	½ cup
Cereal, cold, flake-type	¾ cup
Cereal, granola, low-fat	¼ cup
★ Cereal, hot (with water), unsweetened	½ cup
Corn, canned or frozen	½ cup
★ Corn, fresh	½ cup
Cornbread, from dry mix	1 ounce
★ Corn on the cob	½ large ear
Couscous, cooked	⅓ cup
Crackers, cheese	14 small
Crackers, matzo, whole-wheat	1 cracker (1 ounce)
Crackers, Melba rounds or Melba toast	½ cup or 6 rounds

★   **Blue star indicates the best choices.**

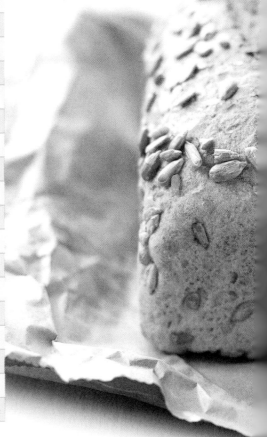

FROM THE DIETITIAN

Carbohydrates are your body's primary fuel supply, and the highest quality fuel comes from whole grains — as well as legumes and fresh fruits and vegetables.

Carbohydrates

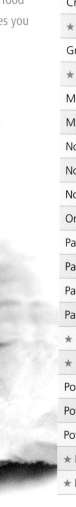

FROM THE DIETITIAN

High-fiber foods are chewier and take longer to eat, so you consume fewer calories. Fiber also slows how quickly food is digested, which makes you feel full longer.

Item (70 calories per serving)	One serving is
Crackers, saltines	5 squares
Crackers, rye	1 triple cracker
Crackers, wheat	8 crackers
Croutons	½ cup
★ English muffin, whole-grain	½
Graham crackers, plain or honey	1 rectangle
★ Kasha (buckwheat or groats), cooked	½ cup
Mixed vegetables, canned or frozen	1 cup
Muffin, any flavor	1 small
Noodles, egg	⅓ cup
Noodles, Japanese (soba)	⅔ cup
Noodles, rice	⅓ cup
Orzo, cooked	¾ cup
Pancake	1 cake (4-inch)
Parsnips	¾ cup
Pasta, macaroni, cooked	⅓ cup
Pasta, spaghetti, cooked	⅓ cup
★ Pasta, whole-grain, cooked	½ cup
★ Pita bread, whole-wheat	½ round (6-inch)
Potatoes, baby, red or white	3
Potatoes, baked	½ medium
Potatoes, mashed	½ cup
★ Pumpkin, cooked	1½ cups
★ Rice, brown, cooked	⅓ cup

★ **Blue star indicates the best choices.**

Carbohydrates

Item (70 calories per serving)	One serving is
Rice, white, cooked	⅓ cup
Rice, wild, cooked	½ cup
★ Rutabaga, cooked	¾ cup
★ Squash, winter, cooked	1 cup
★ Sweet potatoes, baked	½ large
Taco shell, hard	1 medium shell (5-inch)
Tortilla, corn	1 round (6-inch)
★ Turnips, cooked	⅓ cup
Waffle, frozen	1 waffle (4-inch)

★ **Blue star indicates the best choices.**

FROM THE DIETITIAN

Highly refined carbohydrates have had most of their nutrients stripped away during processing. Although some vitamins and minerals may be added back into products, such as white rice and white flour, they still don't have as many other nutrients as whole grains do.

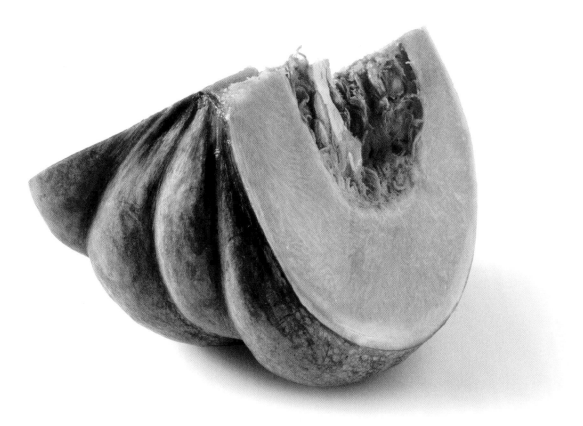

Protein and Dairy

FROM THE DIETITIAN

Proteins are made up of different amino acids, eight of which are called essential because your body can't produce them and they must be obtained via your diet. Common sources of dietary protein include meat, poultry, seafood, eggs, dairy products and legumes.

Item (110 calories per serving)	One serving is
Bacon, Canadian-style	2½ ounces
Beans, baked, canned	½ cup
★ Beans, black	½ cup
★ Beans, chickpeas (garbanzos)	⅓ cup
★ Beans, green soybeans (edamame)	½ cup
★ Beans, kidney	½ cup
★ Beans, navy	¾ cup
Beans, refried, low-fat	½ cup
Beef, ground, regular	2-ounce patty
Beef, ground, 90-95 percent lean	2-ounce patty
Beef, rib-eye steak, trimmed of fat	2 ounces
Beef, sirloin steak, trimmed of fat	2 ounces
Beef, tenderloin, trimmed of fat	2 ounces
Beef jerky	1 ounce
★ Burger, vegetarian	3-ounce patty
Burger crumbles, vegetarian	4 ounces
Cheese, American, fat-free	3 ounces
Cheese, Cheddar or colby, low-fat	2 ounces or ½ cup shredded
Cheese, cottage, low-fat	⅔ cup
Cheese, feta	1½ ounces or ¼ cup
Cheese, Gouda	1 ounce
Cheese, mozzarella, part-skim	1½ ounces or ½ cup shredded
Cheese, Muenster	1 ounce
Cheese, Muenster, low-fat	1½ ounces
Cheese, Parmesan	¼ cup grated

★   **Blue star indicates the best choices.**

Protein and Dairy

Item (110 calories per serving)	One serving is
Cheese, ricotta, part-skim	⅓ cup
Cheese, soybean curd	⅓ cup
Cheese, Swiss	1 ounce
Cheese, Swiss, low-fat	2 ounces
Cheese slice, American, processed	1 ounce
Cheese spread, American	1 ounce
★ Chicken breast, boneless, skinless	2½ ounces
Chicken drumstick, skinless	2½ ounces
Chicken giblets, simmered	2½ ounces or ½ cup
★ Clams, fresh or canned	3 ounces (about 10 small)
★ Crab, fresh, imitation or canned	4 ounces
Duck, breast, skinless, trimmed of fat	2½ ounces
Egg, whole	1 large
Egg substitute, liquid	½ cup
★ Egg whites	1 cup (about 6)
★ Fish, Atlantic salmon, grilled or broiled	2 ounces
★ Fish, cod, grilled or broiled	3 ounces
★ Fish, haddock, grilled or broiled	3 ounces
★ Fish, halibut, grilled or broiled	3 ounces
★ Fish, orange roughy, grilled or broiled	3 ounces
Ham	3 ounces
Lamb, lean, ground	2 ounces
Lamb, lean, trimmed of fat	2 ounces
★ Lentils	½ cup
Lobster, boiled	4 ounces

★   Blue star indicates the best choices.

FROM THE DIETITIAN

Milk and milk products are rich in calcium, potassium and protein, and are often fortified with vitamin D. Choose fat-free or low-fat varieties to keep your blood cholesterol levels healthy.

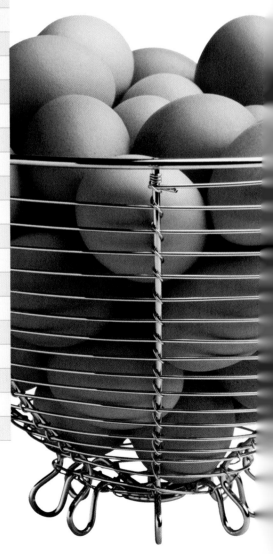

Protein and Dairy

Americans generally consume much more protein than the daily amount recommended by the Food and Drug Administration. Vegetarians may ensure that they're getting enough protein by including lentils, peas, nuts and tofu in their diets.

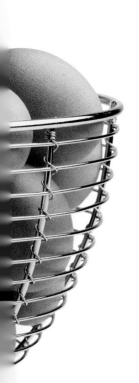

Item (110 calories per serving)	One serving is
Milk, buttermilk, low-fat or reduced-fat	8 ounces or 1 cup
★ Milk, skim or 1%	8 ounces or 1 cup
Mussels	2 ounces
Peas, green, canned	½ cup
Peas, green, fresh or frozen	¾ cup
Pheasant breast, skinless	3 ounces
Pork chops, boneless, trimmed of fat	3 ounces
Pork sausage, smoked	2 small links
Pork tenderloin, roasted, trimmed of fat	3 ounces
★ Scallops	3 ounces
★ Shrimp, fresh or canned	4 ounces
Soy milk, low-fat	8 ounces or 1 cup
Tempeh	2 ounces or ⅓ cup
★ Tofu, firm or silken soft	2 slices (1-inch width)
★ Tuna, fresh or canned in water	3 ounces or ½ cup
Turkey, dark meat, skinless	2 ounces
★ Turkey, white meat, skinless	3 ounces
Turkey breast luncheon meat, fat-free	4 ounces
Turkey meat, ground, cooked	2 ounces
Veal	3 ounces
Venison	3 ounces
★ Yogurt, fat-free, plain, unsweetened or reduced-calorie with fruit	8 ounces or 1 cup
Yogurt, soy, plain, unsweetened	6 ounces or ⅔ cup

★   **Blue star indicates the best choices.**

Fats

Item (45 calories per serving)	One serving is
★ Avocado	⅙ section of fruit
Bacon, pork	1 slice
Bacon, turkey	1 slice
Butter, regular	1 teaspoon
Butter, whipped	1½ teaspoons
Coconut, shredded, sweetened	1½ tablespoons
Cream, heavy	1 tablespoon liquid (4 tablespoons whipped)
Cream cheese, fat-free	3 tablespoons
Cream cheese, regular	1 tablespoon
Creamer, nondairy, flavored	1 tablespoon
Creamer, nondairy, flavored, reduced-fat	1½ tablespoons
Creamer, nondairy, plain	2 tablespoons
Creamer, nondairy, plain, light	2½ tablespoons
Gravy, canned (average of all varieties)	⅓ cup
Guacamole	2 tablespoons
Half-and-half	2 tablespoons
Honey mustard dressing	1½ tablespoons
Margarine, regular or butter-blend	1 teaspoon
Margarine, tub, reduced-fat	1 tablespoon
Margarine, tub, regular	2 teaspoons
Margarine-like spread, light, trans fat-free	1 tablespoon
Margarine-like spread, trans fat-free	2 teaspoons
Mayonnaise, fat-free	4 tablespoons
Mayonnaise, low-calorie	1 tablespoon
Mayonnaise, regular	2 teaspoons

★ **Blue star indicates the best choices.**

FROM THE DIETITIAN

The fact that there's fat in your diet is not the reason why you may be struggling with your weight. You need to eat some fat because it's vital for long life and good health. The problem typically is that people eat too much fat, so choose smaller amounts of healthy fats in your diet.

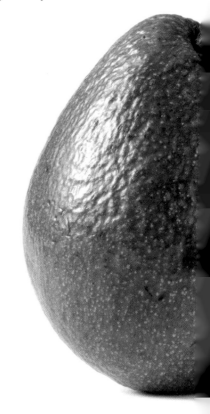

Fats

How you prepare your food can greatly reduce the amount of fat and calories in your diet. Healthy cooking techniques include baking, braising, grilling, broiling, poaching, roasting, sautéing, steaming and stir-frying.

Item (45 calories per serving)	One serving is
★ Nuts, almonds	4 teaspoons slivered or 7 whole
★ Nuts, Brazil	1 whole
★ Nuts, cashew	4 whole
★ Nuts, hickory	2 whole
★ Nuts, peanuts	8 whole
★ Nuts, pecans	4 halves
★ Nuts, walnuts	4 halves
★ Oil, canola	1 teaspoon
Oil, corn	1 teaspoon
★ Oil, olive	1 teaspoon
Oil, peanut	1 teaspoon
Oil, safflower	1 teaspoon
Olives, black or green	9 large or 12 small
Peanut butter, chunky or smooth	1½ teaspoons
Salad dressing, French, fat-free	2 tablespoons
Salad dressing, French, regular	2 teaspoons
Salad dressing, Italian, fat-free	4 tablespoons
Salad dressing, Italian, regular	1 tablespoon
Salad dressing, ranch, fat-free	3 tablespoons
Salad dressing, ranch, regular	2 teaspoons
Salad dressing (mayonnaise-type), fat-free	3 tablespoons
Salad dressing (mayonnaise-type), regular	2 teaspoons
★ Seeds, flaxseed, ground	1 tablespoon

★ **Blue star indicates the best choices.**

Fats

Item (45 calories per serving)	One serving is
★ Seeds, pumpkin	1 tablespoon
★ Seeds, sesame	1 tablespoon
★ Seeds, sunflower	1 tablespoon
Shortening, vegetable	1 teaspoon
Sour cream, fat-free	4 tablespoons
Sour cream, regular	2 tablespoons
Tartar sauce	1 tablespoon
Tartar sauce, low-fat	2 tablespoons
Whipped topping, nondairy	4 tablespoons

★ **Blue star indicates the best choices.**

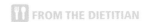

FROM THE DIETITIAN

Monounsaturated fats and polyunsaturated fats — the so-called "healthier" fats — are found in many vegetable oils, fish, olives and nuts. Saturated fats and trans fats are unhealthy and found in many animal-based foods. All types of fats are calorie dense and should be eaten in moderation.

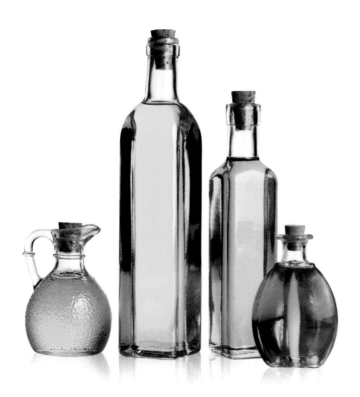

Sweets

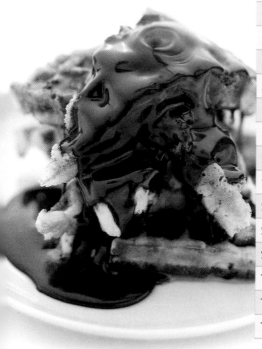

FROM THE DIETITIAN

A craving for sweets is often something you've learned — which means you can also change your taste for sweets by gradually reducing how much sugar you eat and by eating healthier foods.

Item (75 calories per serving)	One serving is
Chocolate chips, semisweet	4 tablespoons
Cranberry sauce, canned, sweetened	3 tablespoons
Frosting, chocolate, ready-to-eat	1 tablespoon
Fruit butter, apple	2½ tablespoons
Gelatin dessert	½ cup
Hard candy (butterscotch, lemon drops, peppermint)	4 pieces
Honey	1 tablespoon
Jellies, jams and preserves (all varieties)	1½ tablespoons
Jellies, jams and preserves, reduced-sugar	4 tablespoons
Jelly beans	20 small or 8 large
Molasses	1½ tablespoons
Rhubarb, cooked and sweetened	¼ cup
Sugar, brown (unpacked)	2 tablespoons
Sugar, granulated, white	4 teaspoons
Sugar, powdered	2 tablespoons
Syrup, light corn	1 tablespoon
Syrup, maple	1½ tablespoons
Topping, butterscotch or caramel	1½ tablespoons
Topping, chocolate syrup	1½ tablespoons
Topping, strawberry	1½ tablespoons

★ **Blue star indicates the best choices.**

Breakfast

Item	Amount	V	F	C	PD	Ft	S
					Food group servings		
Bacon, Canadian-style	2½ ounces				1		
Bacon, fried	1 strip					1	
Bagel, whole-grain	½ bagel (3-inch)			1			
Bagel with egg and cheese	1 sandwich			3	2	1	
Banana	1 small		1				
Biscuit with egg	1 biscuit			2	1	3	
Biscuit with egg and meat	1 biscuit			2	2	2	
Bread, whole-grain	1 slice			1			
Bread, whole-wheat white	1 slice			1			
Cereal, cold, Basic 4-type	⅓ cup			1			
Cereal, cold, shredded wheat, sweetened	¾ cup			1			1
Cereal, cold, bran flakes	½ cup			1			
Croissant, plain	1 medium croissant			2		2	
Croissant with egg and cheese	1 croissant			2	1	2	
Croissant with egg, cheese and bacon	1 croissant			2	1.5	3	
Doughnut, cake (plain)	1 (3¼-inch dia.)			0.5		3	0.5
Doughnut, raised (glazed)	1 (3¾-inch dia.)			1		2	1
Egg, omelet, western	1 large egg	1			1		
Egg, scrambled	1 large egg				1		
English muffin, whole-grain	½ muffin			1			
English muffin with egg, cheese and Canadian bacon	1 muffin			2	1	1	
French toast	1 slice			1	0.5	1	
French toast sticks	5 sticks			2	1	1	1

V **Vegetables**　　C **Carbohydrates**　　Ft **Fats**

F **Fruits**　　PD **Protein/Dairy**　　S **Sweets**

Breakfast

		Food group servings					
Item	**Amount**	**V**	**F**	**C**	**PD**	**Ft**	**S**
Granola, home-prepared	¼ cup			1		2	
Granola, low-fat	¼ cup			1			
Grapefruit	¾ cup sections or ½ large		1				
Hash brown potatoes	½ cup			1.5			3
Melon balls	1 cup (8 balls)		1				
Muffin, blueberry (made with low-fat milk)	1 (2 ounces)			1		1	0.5
Muffin, cranberry-orange	1 large (4 ounces)	0.5		2		4	1
Oatmeal, instant, plain (made with water)	1 packet			1.5			
Oatmeal, instant, sweetened (made with water)	1 packet			1			1
Pancake with berries, syrup and trans-free margarine	1 pancake		1	1		1	1
Pastry, cinnamon Danish	1 (4-inch dia.)			1		3	1
Pastry, cinnamon roll with frosting	1 (2-inch dia.)					1	1
Pastry, toaster-type	1 item			1		2	1
Prunes	3 fruits		1				
Quiche with broccoli and Cheddar cheese	6 ounces	1		0.5	2	4	
Scone with fruit (unfrosted)	1 (4 ounces)			2		4	2
Strawberries	1½ cups whole		1				
Waffle, plain, from recipe	1 (4-inch dia.)			1		1	
Yogurt, plain, low-fat, low-calorie sweetener	1 cup (8 ounces)				1		
Yogurt with fruit, low-fat, low-calorie sweetener	1 cup (8 ounces)				1		

V Vegetables **C** Carbohydrates **Ft** Fats
F Fruits **PD** Protein/Dairy **S** Sweets

Sandwich

		Food group servings					
Item	**Amount**	**V**	**F**	**C**	**PD**	**Ft**	**S**
Bacon, lettuce and tomato	1 sandwich	1		2		4	
Cheeseburger, single patty with condiments	1 sandwich			3	2	2	
Chicken, grilled	1 sandwich	1		2	1		
Chicken cordon bleu, restaurant-prepared	1 sandwich			3	2.5	2	
Chicken fillet, grilled, with mayonnaise	1 sandwich			3	2	2	
Chicken wrap	1 wrap	1	1	1	1		1
Fish, with tartar sauce	1 sandwich			3	1.5	1	
French dip, restaurant-prepared	1 sandwich			4	2	1	
Ham and cheese, hot	1 sandwich			2	1.5	1	
Ham and cheese, stuffed pocket, microwave	1 sandwich			3	3	3	
Hamburger, California (vegetables, mayonnaise)	1 sandwich	1		2	2	1	
Hamburger, single patty with condiments	1 sandwich			2	1	1	
Hot dog (frankfurter), beef	1½-ounce dog			2	1	1	
Peanut butter and jelly	1 sandwich			2		2	1
Roast beef, plain, restaurant-prepared	1 regular			2	1.5	1	
Steak	1 sandwich			2	2		
Submarine with cold cuts	about 6 inches	1		3	1.5	1	
Submarine with tuna salad	about 6 inches	1		3	2	3	
Tuna salad pita	1 sandwich			1	1	1	
Turkey (vegetables, mayonnaise)	1 sandwich	1		2	1	1	
Turkey ranch and bacon, restaurant-prepared	1 sandwich	3		4	3	3	
Turkey wrap, smoked	1 wrap			1	1	1	

V Vegetables **C** Carbohydrates **Ft** Fats
F Fruits **PD** Protein/Dairy **S** Sweets

Salad and Soup

Item	Amount	V	F	C	PD	Ft	S
Salad							
Caesar salad with grilled chicken	11 ounces	3			1	1	
Coleslaw, home-prepared	1 cup	2					1
Potato salad, home-prepared	1 cup	1		2		4	
Spinach salad with fruit	1 salad	2	1				1
Taco salad (fast food)	1½ cups	1		1	1	2	
Tossed salad with cheese and egg, no dressing	2 cups	2			1.5		
Tossed salad with pasta and seafood, no dressing	1½ cups	2		1	2	1	
Tossed salad with turkey, ham and cheese, no dressing	1½ cups	2			2		
Soup or stew							
Bean with pork, canned (made with water)	1 cup			1	1		
Beef stew, canned	1 cup	2		0.5	1	1	
Broccoli, cream of, canned (made with low-fat milk)	1 cup	1			1		
Chicken noodle, canned (broth-based)	1 cup			1			
Chilie con carne, with beans	1 cup	1			2		
Clam chowder, New England, canned	1 cup				1.5		
Hot and sour	1 cup			0.5	0.5		
Miso (from 1 tablespoon of miso)	1 cup				0.5		
Mushroom, cream of, canned (made with water)	1 cup				1		
Split pea with ham, canned (made with water)	1 cup				2		
Tomato or tomato-based, canned (made with water)	1 cup			1			
Vegetable or vegetable beef, canned (broth-based)	1 cup			1			

V **Vegetables**　　C **Carbohydrates**　　Ft **Fats**
F **Fruits**　　PD **Protein/Dairy**　　S **Sweets**

Main Course

Item	Amount				Food group servings					
		V	F	C	PD	Ft	S
Beef, round roast	2 ounces				1		
Beef, sirloin steak, trimmed of fat	2 ounces				1		
Burrito, beef, beans and cheese	1 burrito			1	2	1	
Burrito, chicken, supreme	1 burrito	1		2	1.5	3	
Chicken, dark meat, fried (fast food)	2 pieces			1	2.5	2	
Chicken, white meat, fried (fast food)	2 pieces			1	3	2	
Chicken breast or drumstick, grilled	2½ ounces				1		
Chicken patty, breaded and fried (fast food)	3-ounce patty			1	1	2	
Chicken stir-fry	1 entree	3		1	1		
Crab cake, breaded and fried	3-ounce cake			0.5	1	2	
Fajitas, beef, pork or chicken	2 fajitas	2		2	1	1	
Fish, cod, haddock or halibut, grilled or broiled	3-ounce fillet				1		
Fish fillet, breaded and fried	3-ounce fillet			1	1	1	
Fish sticks, breaded and fried	3 sticks			1	1	1	
Lasagna with meat	2½-x-4-inch piece	2		1	1.5	1	
Kebabs, beef	1 skewer	2			2		
Kebabs, chicken	1 skewer	2			1		
Kielbasa, Polish, smoked	3 ounces				1	2	
Macaroni and cheese, from mix	1 cup			2	2	1	
Meatballs, Swedish with cream or white sauce	1 cup (about 5 meatballs)			1	2	2	
Meatloaf, lean ground beef	3-ounce slice	1			1	1	
Pasta primavera	1 entree	2		2	1	1	

V	Vegetables	C	Carbohydrates	Ft	Fats
F	Fruits	PD	Protein/Dairy	S	Sweets

Main Course

Item	Amount	Food group servings					
		V	F	C	PD	Ft	S
Pizza, cheese, regular crust	⅛ of 14-inch	1		1	1	1	
Pizza, cheese, regular crust, frozen	⅓ of 12-inch	2		2	1	2	
Pizza, pepperoni, regular crust	⅛ of 14-inch	1		1.5	1	1	
Pizza, pepperoni, regular crust, frozen	⅓ of 12-inch	2		2	1.5	2	
Pizza, pepperoni, thick crust	⅛ of 14-inch	1		2	1	1	
Pork chops, boneless, trimmed of fat	3 ounces				1		
Pork ribs, country-style, lean	2½ ounces				1	2	
Pork tenderloin, roasted, trimmed of fat	3 ounces				1		
Potpie, beef, frozen	1 pie (9 ounces)	2		2	1	3	
Potpie, chicken or turkey, frozen	1 pie (9 ounces)	2		2	1	3	
Shrimp, breaded and fried	4 ounces			1	1	2	
Skillet meal, "helper," with lean ground beef, chicken or tuna	1 cup	1		1	1.5	1	
Spaghetti with meatballs and tomato sauce, canned	1 cup	2		2	0.5	1	
Spaghetti with marinara sauce	1 cup	2		2		1	
Taco, beef or chicken, hard shell	1 taco	1		1	0.5	1	
Taco with beef, soft shell	1 taco	1		1	0.5	1	
Tortellini with cheese filling	¾ cup			2	2		

V Vegetables	**C** Carbohydrates	**Ft** Fats
F Fruits	**PD** Protein/Dairy	**S** Sweets

Side Dish

Item	Amount	V	F	C	PD	Ft	S
Beans, baked, with pork, franks or beef, canned	1 cup			1	2	1	
Biscuit (fast food)	1 large			2		2	
Bread, garlic	1 slice			1		1	
Breadstick, soft (fast food)	1 stick			1		1	
Buffalo wings	4 pieces				1	2	
Chicken tenders	4 pieces			1	1	1	
Chow mein noodles	⅓ cup			0.5	1		
Crescent roll, from refrigerated dough	1 roll			1		1	
Egg rolls, vegetable, chicken or pork	3-ounce roll	1		1	0.5		
French fries	1 small serving			2		2	
Hummus, home-prepared	4 tablespoons			1			
Mozzarella sticks, deep-fried (fast food)	4 sticks			1	2	3	
Onion rings, breaded (fast food)	8-9 rings	2		1.5		3	
Potato, baked, with cheese and broccoli (fast food)	1 potato	1		3	1	2	
Potato, mashed, with gravy	about ½ cup			1.5		1	
Potatoes, au gratin, with trans-free margarine	½ cup			1	0.5	1	
Potatoes, scalloped, with trans-free margarine	½ cup			1		0.5	
Salsa	¼ cup	1					
Tortilla, flour	1 round (6-inch)			1		.5	

V Vegetables	**C** Carbohydrates	**Ft** Fats
F Fruits	**PD** Protein/Dairy	**S** Sweets

Snack

Item	Amount	V	F	C	PD	Ft	S
Bread, banana	1 slice	0.5	1			1	1
Cereal bar, granola-type or fruit filled	1 bar			1			1
Cheese puff or twist	1 ounce			1		2	
Chex mix or oriental mix	½ cup			1		1	
Cracker, sandwich, with peanut butter filling	6 crackers			1.5		2	
Fruit leather pieces	1 pack (¾ ounces)		1				
Popcorn, microwave, buttered	3 cups			1		2	
Popcorn, plain, air popped	3 cups			1			
Popcorn, plain, oil popped	3 cups			1		2	
Potato chips	1 ounce			1		2	
Potato chips, baked	1 ounce			1		1	
Pretzel sticks, small	about 30			1			
Pretzel twists	about 3			1			
Rice cakes, most types	2 cakes			1			
Soybeans, dry roasted	2 tablespoons				1		
Strawberry smoothie	1 smoothie		1		1		
Tortilla chips or corn chips, baked	1 ounce			1		1	
Tortilla chips or corn chips, regular	1 ounce			1		2	
Trail mix, with chocolate chips, nuts and seeds	½ cup					5	2
Yogurt, fat-free, plain, unsweetened or reduced-calorie with fruit	8 ounces or 1 cup				1		

Food group servings

V	Vegetables	C	Carbohydrates	Ft	Fats
F	Fruits	PD	Protein/Dairy	S	Sweets

Dessert

		Food group servings					
Item	**Amount**	V	F	C	PD	Ft	S
Bar, brownie	3-inch square			1		2	1
Bar, lemon	1½-ounce bar					1	1.5
Cake, angel food	¹⁄₁₂ of 12-ounce cake						1
Cake, chocolate, no frosting	¹⁄₁₂ of 9-inch diameter cake			1		3	2
Cake, cinnamon, with crumb topping	⅛ of 8-x-6-inch cake			1		1	1
Cake, gingerbread	⅑ of 8-x-8-inch cake			1		3	1
Cake, pound, fat-free	1-ounce slice						1
Cake, white, no frosting	¹⁄₁₂ of 9-inch diameter cake			1.5		2	1
Chocolate bar, milk	1 bar (1½ ounces)					2	1.5
Chocolate bar, dark	1 ounce					2	1
Cookie, chocolate chip	2 medium					1	0.5
Cookie, chocolate sandwich with creme filling	2 standard					1	1
Cookie, fig bar	2 standard		.5			1	0.5
Cookie, gingersnap	3 medium						1
Cookie, oatmeal raisin, peanut butter or sugar	1 3-inch cookie						1
Custard	½ cup				0.5		1
Ice cream, light (average of most flavors)	½ cup					1	1
Ice cream, regular (average of most flavors)	½ cup					2	0.5
Ice cream, soft serve, vanilla, light	½ cup					1	1

V **Vegetables**   C **Carbohydrates**   Ft **Fats**
F **Fruits**   PD **Protein/Dairy**   S **Sweets**

Dessert

Item	Amount	V	F	C	PD	Ft	S
					Food group servings		
Juice bar, frozen	1 bar (3 ounces)		1				
Pudding, instant, sugar-sweetened, 2% milk	½ cup				0.5	0.5	1
Pudding, tapioca, sugar-sweetened, 2% milk	½ cup				0.5	0.5	1
Shake, vanilla or chocolate (fast food)	12 fluid ounces				2		2
Sherbet and sorbet	⅓ cup						1
Pie, chocolate creme, commercially prepared	⅛ of 9-inch diameter pie			1	1	4	1
Pie, fruit, (apple, blueberry or cherry), from recipe	⅛ of 9-inch diameter pie		1	1		4	1
Pie, lemon meringue, commercially prepared	⅙ of 8-inch diameter pie	0.5	0.5			2	2
Pie, pecan	⅛ of 9-inch diameter pie			1	1	4	2
Pie, pumpkin	⅛ of 9-inch diameter pie	1		1		3	1
Yogurt, frozen, fat-free	½ cup				0.5		1

V **Vegetables**   C **Carbohydrates**   Ft **Fats**
F **Fruits**   PD **Protein/Dairy**   S **Sweets**

Healthy dessert ›
See page 245 for the recipe for Blueberry and Lemon Cream Parfait.

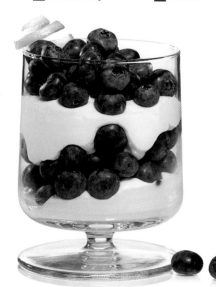

Beverage

		Food group servings					
Item	**Amount**	V	F	C	PD	Ft	S
Alcohol							
Beer, light	12 fluid ounces						1.5
Beer, regular	12 fluid ounces						2
Distilled spirits (gin, rum, vodka, whiskey)	1 fluid ounce						1
Wine, red or white	5 fluid ounces						1.5
Coffee or tea drinks							
Caffe latte or caffe mocha, skim	12 fluid ounces				1		
Cappuccino	12 fluid ounces				0.5		
Chai tea, with skim milk	12 fluid ounces				1		1
Coffee, brewed or instant	8 fluid ounces			calorie-free beverage			
Tea, iced, commercially sweetened	12 fluid ounces						2
Tea, regular or herbal, brewed or instant	8 fluid ounces			calorie-free beverage			
Dairy or cocoa drinks							
Chocolate-flavored mix, made with low-fat milk	8 fluid ounces				1		1
Chocolate milk, made with skim or 1% milk	8 fluid ounces				1		0.5
Cocoa, hot, made with water	6 fluid ounces				0.5		0.5
Milk, 2% or whole	8 fluid ounces				1	1	
Fruit-flavored drinks							
Fruit punch, from powder	8 fluid ounces						1.5
Lemonade, from sweetened concentrate	8 fluid ounces		1				0.5
Orange breakfast drink, ready-to-serve	8 fluid ounces						1.5

V Vegetables	**C** Carbohydrates	**Ft** Fats
F Fruits	**PD** Protein/Dairy	**S** Sweets

Beverage

Item	Amount	Food group servings					
		V	F	C	PD	Ft	S
Juices							
Cranberry, sweetened	4 fluid ounces		1				
Orange, grapefruit or pineapple, unsweetened	4 fluid ounces		1				
Tomato or vegetable	4 fluid ounces	1					
Soft drinks							
Club soda	12 fluid ounces	calorie-free beverage					
Cola, lemon-lime or root beer, regular	12 fluid ounces						2
Cream soda, regular	12 fluid ounces						2.5
Diet soda, any flavor	12 fluid ounces	calorie-free beverage					
Ginger ale, regular	12 fluid ounces						1.5
Sports drink							
Fruit-flavored, ready-to-drink, low-calorie	12 fluid ounces						0.5
Fruit-flavored, ready-to-drink, regular	12 fluid ounces						1
Adding calories to your coffee and tea							
Cream, heavy	1 tablespoon					1	
Creamer, nondairy, flavored	1 tablespoon					1	
Creamer, nondairy, plain	2 tablespoons					1	
Creamer, nondairy, plain, light	2½ tablespoons					1	
Half-and-half	2 tablespoons					1	
Sugar	2 teaspoons						0.5

V Vegetables	**C** Carbohydrates	**Ft** Fats
F Fruits	**PD** Protein/Dairy	**S** Sweets

Recipes
for weight loss

Can you lose weight and eat well at the same time? Of
course! The menu decisions you make each day should be
based on a variety of foods and kitchen techniques
that can help keep you healthy. The recipes that
follow show how easy and enjoyable eating
well can be.

Baked Chicken With Pears

10 MINUTES PREPARATION TIME ✛ 20 MINUTES COOKING TIME ✛ SERVES 8

8	4-oz. boneless, skinless chicken breasts
1	tsp. tarragon
1	tbsp. olive oil (divided)
4	medium sweet onions, thinly sliced
4	pears, seeded and thinly sliced
1	c. low-fat feta cheese crumbles

1. Preheat oven to 375 F.
2. Rub each chicken breast with tarragon.
3. In a large, ovenproof skillet, heat ½ tablespoon olive oil and cook chicken 2 to 3 minutes a side until lightly golden. Add remaining oil and sliced onion and continue to cook until onions are translucent.
4. Lightly cover the skillet with foil. Place skillet in oven and bake chicken and onions about 15 minutes. Chicken should reach 165 F when tested with a meat thermometer. Remove from oven. Let rest (still covered) about 5 minutes before serving.
5. Plate chicken as follows: Make a bed of cooked onion, place chicken on top. Arrange pear slices on and around chicken. Sprinkle each with 2 table-spoons feta. Serve.

PYRAMID SERVINGS:

V	Vegetables	3
F	Fruits	1
PD	Protein/Dairy	1

PER SERVING

Calories	255
Protein	31 g
Carbohydrate	26 g
Total fat	3 g
Monounsaturated fat	1.6 g
Cholesterol	66 mg
Sodium	199 mg
Fiber	4 g

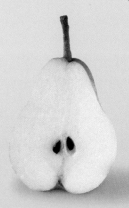

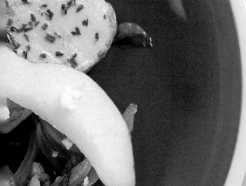

Breakfast Burrito

5 MINUTES PREPARATION TIME + 10 MINUTES COOKING TIME + SERVES 1

½ c. chopped tomato

2 tbsp. chopped onion

¼ c. canned corn — with no salt added

¼ c. egg substitute

1 whole-wheat flour tortilla, 6-inch diameter

2 tbsp. salsa

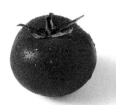

1. In a small skillet, add the chopped tomato, onion and corn. Cook over medium heat until the vegetables are soft and moisture is evaporated.

2. Add the egg substitute and scramble with the vegetables until cooked through, about 3 minutes.

3. Spread the egg mixture in the center of the tortilla and top with salsa. Fold both sides of the tortilla up over the filling, then roll to close. Serve immediately.

PYRAMID SERVINGS:

V	Vegetables	1
C	Carbohydrates	2
PD	Protein/Dairy	.5

PER SERVING

Calories	231
Protein	12 g
Carbohydrate	34 g
Total fat	5 g
Monounsaturated fat	2 g
Cholesterol	1 mg
Sodium	519 mg
Fiber	8 g

Heart-Healthy Oatmeal

5 MINUTES PREPARATION TIME + 10 MINUTES COOKING TIME + SERVES 6

3¼ c. water

2 c. old-fashioned rolled oats

1 c. blueberries

¼ c. dried cranberries or raisins

¼ c. brown sugar

2 c. fat-free vanilla yogurt, sweetened with low-calorie sweetener

¼ c. chopped walnuts

1. In a medium saucepan, bring water to a boil; stir in oats. Return to a boil and reduce heat to medium. Cook about 5 minutes or until most of the liquid is absorbed. Stir frequently. Remove from heat.

2. Mix fruit into oatmeal. Spoon into bowls. Top with brown sugar, yogurt and walnuts. Serve.

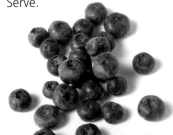

PYRAMID SERVINGS:

F	Fruits	1
C	Carbohydrates	1
PD	Protein/Dairy	.5
Ft	Fats	1
S	Sweets	1

PER SERVING

Calories	249
Protein	9 g
Carbohydrate	42 g
Total fat	5 g
Monounsaturated fat	2 g
Cholesterol	1 mg
Sodium	51 mg
Fiber	5 g

Morning Glory Muffins

15 MINUTES PREPARATION TIME + **35 MINUTES COOKING TIME** + **MAKES 18 SMALL MUFFINS**

1	c. all-purpose (plain) flour
1	c. whole-wheat flour
¾	c. sugar
2	tsp. baking soda
2	tsp. ground cinnamon
¼	tsp. salt
¾	c. egg substitute
½	c. vegetable oil
½	c. unsweetened applesauce
2	tsp. vanilla extract
2	c. chopped apples, unpeeled
½	c. raisins
¾	c. grated carrots
2	tbsp. chopped pecans

1. Preheat the oven to 350 F.
2. Line a muffin pan with paper or foil liners.
3. In a bowl, combine the flours, sugar, baking soda, cinnamon and salt. Whisk to blend evenly.
4. In a separate bowl, add egg substitute, oil, applesauce and vanilla. Stir in apples, raisins and carrots. Add to the flour mixture and blend just until moistened but still slightly lumpy.
5. Spoon the batter into muffin cups, filling each cup about ⅔ full. Sprinkle with chopped pecans and bake until springy to the touch, about 35 minutes.
6. Let cool for 5 minutes, then transfer the muffins to a wire rack and let cool completely. Serve.

PYRAMID SERVINGS:

F	Fruits	1
C	Carbohydrates	1
Ft	Fats	1

PER SERVING (1 MUFFIN)

Calories	170
Protein	3 g
Carbohydrate	25 g
Total fat	7 g
Monounsaturated fat	2 g
Saturated fat	1 g
Cholesterol	trace
Sodium	195 mg
Fiber	2 g

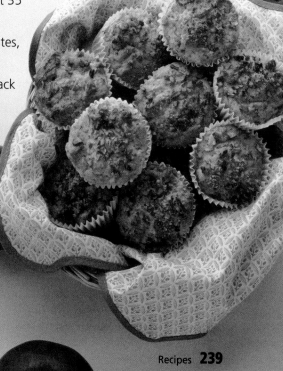

Bulgur Salad With Fruits and Nuts

15 MINUTES PREPARATION TIME + **30 MINUTES COOKING TIME** + **SERVES 8**

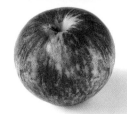

1 c. raw bulgur

2 c. boiling water

⅔ c. coarsely chopped walnuts

½ c. raisins or currants

1 large rib celery, finely diced

¼ c. toasted sunflower seeds

2 tbsp. chives, minced

1 medium apple

juice of half a lemon

¼ c. olive oil

2 tbsp. honey

½ tsp. cumin

¼ tsp. cinnamon

dash of nutmeg

1. Place the bulgur in a heat-proof mixing bowl and pour 2 cups boiling water over it. Cover the bowl and let it stand for 30 minutes, or until the water is absorbed.
2. Fluff with a fork.
3. In a serving bowl, combine the walnuts, raisins, celery, sunflower seeds and chives.
4. Core (but don't peel) the apple and dice it finely. Toss it with the lemon juice in a small bowl.
5. Add apple, along with the remaining ingredients, to the nut-raisin mixture. Stir well.
6. Stir in the bulgur.
7. Serve at once, or chill until needed.

PYRAMID SERVINGS:

F	Fruits	1
C	Carbohydrates	1
Ft	Fats	3

PER SERVING

Calories	246
Protein	5 g
Carbohydrate	26 g
Total fat	14 g
Monounsaturated fat	7 g
Saturated fat	2 g
Polyunsaturated fat	5 g
Cholesterol	0 mg
Sodium	9 mg
Fiber	5 g

This recipe is one of 400 collected in *Fix-It and Enjoy-It! Healthy Cookbook* published by Good Books and available in bookstores.

Dietitian's tip:
All walnuts are high in phosphorus, zinc, copper, iron, potassium, and vitamin E and low in saturated fat. English walnuts have twice as many omega-3 fatty acids — which are good for heart health — as do black walnuts.

Chill out!
The bulgur salad tastes better if it stands awhile, chilled, so the flavors can mix.

Simple Spaghetti With Marinara Sauce

10 MINUTES PREPARATION TIME ✛ 45 TO 90 MINUTES COOKING TIME ✛ SERVES 8

1 large onion, chopped

2 garlic cloves, minced (or more according to preference)

1 tbsp. olive oil

2 28-oz. cans of whole, peeled tomatoes and juice — with no salt added

¼ c. parsley, chopped

12 oz. uncooked whole-wheat spaghetti

2 oz. finely grated Parmesan cheese (about ¾ c.)

1. In a large skillet, cook onions and garlic in olive oil over medium heat until soft. Add tomatoes, including juice, and parsley. Simmer, breaking up tomatoes into smaller pieces. (To make thicker sauce, simmer for up to 1½ hours.)

2. Fill a large pot ¾ full with water. Bring to a boil. Add the spaghetti and cook until "al dente" or until tender, yet with texture. (See package directions for time.) Drain pasta thoroughly.

3. In a large heated bowl, combine the spaghetti and sauce. Toss gently to mix. Serve — each serving topped with Parmesan cheese.

PYRAMID SERVINGS:

V	Vegetables	2
C	Carbohydrates	2
Ft	Fats	1

PER SERVING

Calories	247
Protein	10 g
Carbohydrate	43 g
Total fat	5 g
Monounsaturated fat	2 g
Saturated fat	1.5 g
Cholesterol	5 mg
Sodium	140 mg
Fiber	7 g

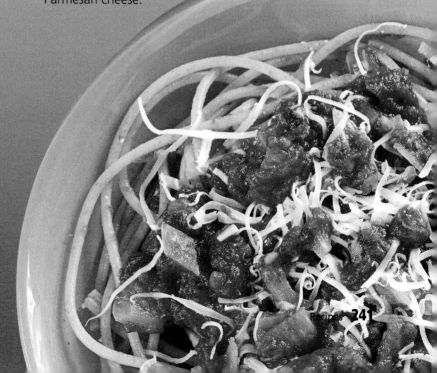

Brown Rice With Vegetables

15 MINUTES PREPARATION TIME ✛ 45 MINUTES COOKING TIME ✛ SERVES 8

1 c. brown rice, uncooked

1 tbsp. olive oil

2 c. reduced-sodium chicken broth (or water)

4 scallions (green onions including tops)

2 c. total — chopped red, green or yellow bell peppers, celery, mushrooms, asparagus, peapods or carrots

2 tbsp. lemon juice

Optional: ground black pepper, chopped fresh parsley

1. In a large saucepan, over medium heat, sauté the rice in oil for about 2 minutes stirring frequently. Reduce heat, slowly add broth, and simmer covered without stirring or opening the lid for about 30 minutes.

2. In the meantime, chop scallions including green tops into small pieces. Do the same with your choice of vegetables.

3. When rice has cooked 30 minutes, add the vegetables and lemon juice. Stir well to combine. Cover pan and continue to cook over medium heat until rice is tender but still has some texture (about 10 to 15 minutes more).

4. Season with black pepper and top with chopped fresh parsley (if desired) and serve.

PYRAMID SERVINGS:

V	Vegetables	1
C	Carbohydrates	1
Ft	Fats	1

PER SERVING

Calories	141
Protein	3 g
Carbohydrate	21 g
Total fat	3 g
Monounsaturated fat	1.5 g
Cholesterol	1 mg
Sodium	44 mg
Fiber	2 g

Grilled Salmon With Sliced Cucumber and Radish

15 MINUTES PREPARATION TIME ✦ 8 TO 10 MINUTES COOKING TIME ✦ SERVES 8

2   lbs. salmon fillet

1   tsp. lemon juice

1   tbsp. olive oil

2   c. cucumber, seeded and thinly sliced

¾   c. radishes, thinly sliced

2   tbsp. vinegar

¼   tsp. dill weed

Optional: ground black pepper

1. Rub salmon with lemon juice, then 1 tsp. of oil. Sprinkle with black pepper, if desired. Cut into 8 pieces. Place salmon, skin side down, onto aluminum foil sprayed with cooking spray.
2. In a bowl, combine the remaining ingredients. Mix well and refrigerate.
3. Grill or broil at medium to high heat until salmon is flaky but still moist. (For best results use a food thermometer. The internal temperature should be 145 F.)
4. Top each serving of salmon with the cucumber and radish mixture.

PYRAMID SERVINGS:

V	Vegetables	1
PD	Protein/Dairy	1
Ft	Fats	1

PER SERVING

Calories	168
Protein	23 g
Carbohydrate	1 g
Total fat	8 g
Monounsaturated fat	3 g
Cholesterol	62 mg
Sodium	54 mg
Fiber	trace

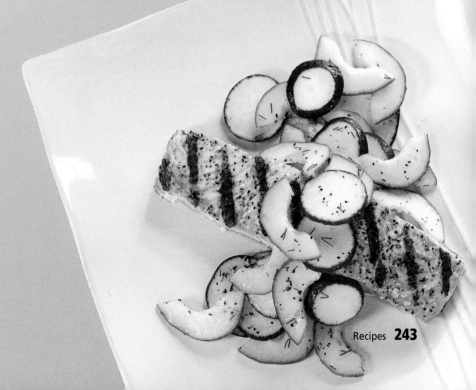

Shrimp Stir-Fry

10 MINUTES PREPARATION TIME ✚ 8 TO 10 MINUTES COOKING TIME ✚ SERVES 4

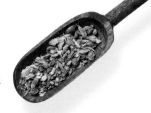

1-2 cloves garlic, chopped

⅛ tsp. fresh ginger, grated or finely chopped,

1 tbsp. olive oil

2½ c. (about ½ lb.) fresh sugar snap peas

½ c. red bell sweet pepper, chopped (optional)

12 oz. medium-sized raw shrimp, peeled and deveined

1. Sauté garlic and ginger in oil in large skillet until fragrant.
2. Stir in peas, and chopped bell pepper if desired. Sauté until tender-crisp.
3. Stir in shrimp. Cook over medium heat 3 to 4 minutes until shrimp are just opaque in centers.
4. Serve with steamed rice (not included in nutrition analysis).

PYRAMID SERVINGS:

V Vegetables	1
PD Protein/Dairy	1
Ft Fats	.5

PER SERVING

Calories	156
Protein	19 g
Carbohydrate	8 g
Total fat	5 g
Monounsaturated fat	2.5 g
Saturated fat	0.7 g
Polyunsaturated fat	5 g
Cholesterol	129 mg
Sodium	136 mg
Fiber	2 g

This recipe is one of 400 collected in *Fix-It and Enjoy-It! Healthy Cookbook* published by Good Books and available in bookstores.

▲ **Portion size**
See page 86 in chapter 8 for a demonstation of how to estimate pyramid servings for this recipe.

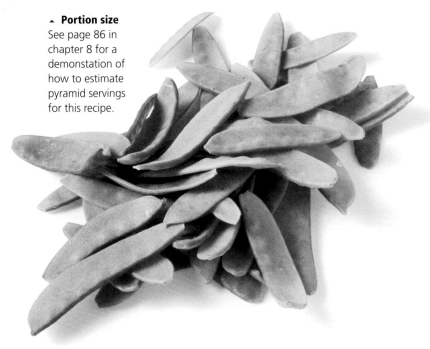

Blueberry and Lemon Cream Parfait

10 MINUTES PREPARATION TIME + SERVES 4

6 oz. low-fat, vanilla yogurt sweetened with low-calorie sweetener

4 oz. fat-free cream cheese

1 tsp. honey

2 tsp. freshly grated lemon zest

3 c. fresh blueberries, rinsed and drained well

1. Drain liquid from the yogurt. In a medium bowl, combine the yogurt, cream cheese and honey. Use an electric mixer to beat at high speed until the yogurt mixture is light and creamy.

2. Stir the lemon zest into the mixture.

3. Layer the lemon cream and blueberries in dessert dishes.

4. Serve at once, or cover and refrigerate until needed.

PYRAMID SERVINGS:

F	Fruits	1
PD	Protein/Dairy	.5

PER SERVING

Calories	125
Protein	7 g
Carbohydrate	22 g
Total fat	1 g
Monounsaturated fat	trace
Cholesterol	4 mg
Sodium	180 mg
Fiber	3 g

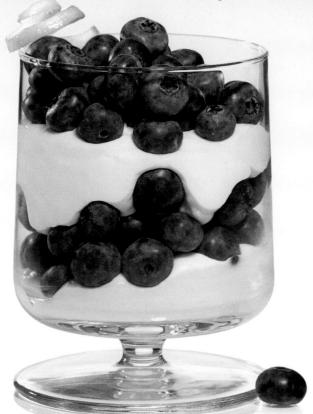

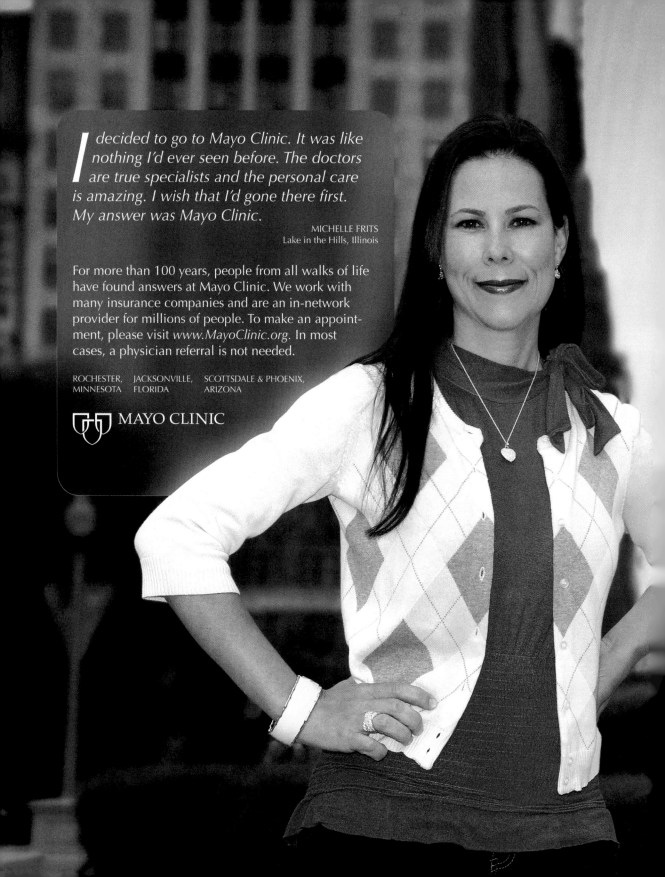

Index

nutrition obstacles *(cont.)*
  menu planning difficulty, 189
  no cooking enjoyment, 182
  skipping breakfast, 188
  travel, 187
  vegetable and fruit dislike, 183

O

obesity
  body mass index (BMI), 110
  disease risk and, 109

overweight, reasons for, 110–111

P

physical activity, 30–31, 131
  adding, 91, 96
  aerobic, 97
  defined, 92
  intensity, 48, 93, 97
  key points, 173
  measurement, 97
  records, 48–49, 95–97
  starting, 31, 94–95
  tiredness and exercise, 191

physical activity obstacles
  age, 193
  arthritis, 197
  embarrassment, 195
  exercise dislike, 192
  exercise environment, 194
  time, 190
  travel, 196

plateaus, 143

portion control, 70, 81
  breakfast, 82–83
  dinner, 86–88
  lunch, 84–85

portions
  defined, 80
  servings vs., 71–72

positive, accentuating, 146–147

protein, 115, 128–129
  as calorie source, 117
  defined, 117
  in food stock, 159
  servings, 217–219
  sources, 128–129

pyramid. *See* Mayo Clinic Healthy Weight
  Pyramid

Q

quick & healthy menu ideas, 161

quick reference guide, Lose It!, 19

R

readiness assessment, 15–17

recipes
  Baked Chicken With Pears, 237
  Blueberry and Lemon Cream Parfait, 245
  Breakfast Burrito, 238
  Brown Rice With Vegetables, 242
  Bulgur Salad With Fruit and Nuts, 240
  Grilled Salmon With Cucumber and Radish,
    243
  Heart-Healthy Oatmeal, 238
  Morning Glory Muffins, 239
  Shrimp Stir-Fry, 244
  Simple Spaghetti With Marinara Sauce, 241
  substitutions in, 164

records
  activity, 48–49, 95–97
  food, 46–47, 138
  overview of, 45

relapses, 144

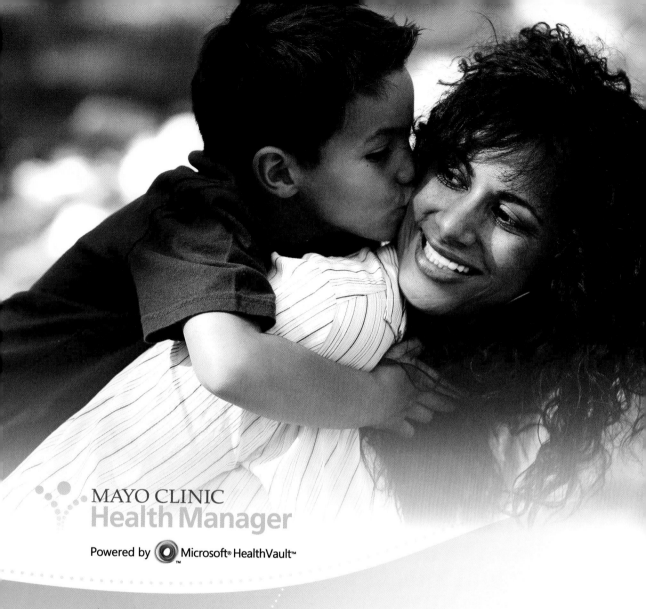

Stay on the path to a healthy new you!

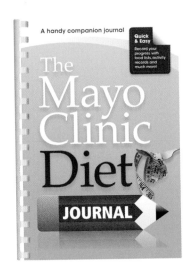

You made a wise decision when you purchased *The Mayo Clinic Diet* book. Here's additional and vital help ... *The Mayo Clinic Diet Journal.* This essential companion to the book allows you to plan, record and journal the new lifestyle habits you've begun and helps you stay on track to a healthier you.

See the ordering information below and place your order today!

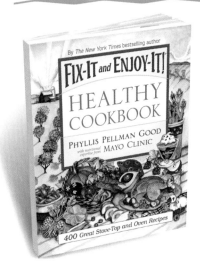

400 quick, healthy and delicious recipes
— from *The New York Times* best-selling cookbook author Phyllis Pellman Good and Mayo Clinic!

Discover the best of both worlds — easy and delicious recipes with special attention to health benefits. Each and every one of the 400 recipes in this book relies heavily on ingredients that are rich in nutrients considered to promote health and prevent disease. Plus, each recipe has been analyzed by Mayo Clinic dietitians for nutritional value and adapted to fit within the *Mayo Clinic Healthy Weight Pyramid.*

To order these and other Mayo Clinic books, newsletters and DVDs — visit us online or call our toll-free number:

Bookstore.MayoClinic.com
877-647-6397

Available from bookstores everywhere, or order from the publisher:

GoodBooks.com
800-762-7171, ext. 221

When you purchase Mayo Clinic books, DVDs and newsletters, proceeds are used to further medical education and research at Mayo Clinic.